Water Exercises
for Rheumatoid Arthritis

Water Exercises

for

Rheumatoid Arthritis

The Effective Way to Reduce Pain and Inflammation While Increasing Flexibility and Mobility

Ann A. Rosenstein

Idyll Arbor, Inc.   Enumclaw, WA

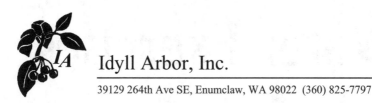

Idyll Arbor, Inc.

39129 264th Ave SE, Enumclaw, WA 98022 (360) 825-7797

Idyll Arbor, Inc. Editor: Thomas M. Blaschko

Photographs: Leroy Cech

Library of Congress Cataloging-in-Publication Data
Rosenstein, Ann A., 1958-
  Water exercises for rheumatoid arthritis : the effective way to reduce pain and inflammation while increasing flexibility and mobility / Ann A. Rosenstein.
      p. cm.
  Includes bibliographical references and index.
  ISBN 978-1-882883-63-9 (alk. paper)
  1. Rheumatoid arthritis--Exercise therapy. 2. Aquatic exercises--Therapeutic use. 3. Rheumatoid arthritis--Patients--Rehabilitation. I. Title.
  RC933.R665 2008
  616.7'2270642--dc22

                                            2008000657

ISBN 1-882883-63-2, 9781882883639

DEDICATION

To my mother and father
Freda and Richard Hosen.
Thank you for being great parents.

Contents

ACKNOWLEDGMENTS

It gives me great pleasure to thank the many people who helped put this book together. First I would like to express my sincere thanks and appreciation to my husband Leo who offered important suggestions, insights, and computer support. To Leroy Cech, my photographer, whose critical eye for detail is revealed in the pictures throughout the book. To Ed Mako who took time to help edit this project in its early stages and to the Lifetime Fitness Club in Burnsville, MN for allowing me to use their pool and pool equipment.

I am also grateful to all the people who took the time to carefully pose for the many illustrations presented. They are Dinah Harlow, Mary Anne Auwarter, Beth Twedten, Leo Rosenstein, Richard Dick, Leroy Cech, and Ed Mako.

Lastly, I would like to thank my editor Thomas Blaschko for his expertise and hard work.

Foreword

Aquatic therapists, aquatic practitioners, and clients all need specific, well-researched, quality guidance to lead those with rheumatoid arthritis toward better physical health and general wellness. Many of the technical manuals available are written for general health. Many other manuals provide great information on specific techniques. Other resources are available only for those who attended workshops. The time has come when books like this are finally available and accessible to serve the specific need of those with RA and those that help them.

The Aquatic Exercise and Therapy Services Industry has made great strides in creating a network that provides education and resources to support the growth and improvement of aquatic services. This book is a reflection of the successful effort to better serve those with chronic disease by telling them that water has magical healing properties. It puts together a good base of theory, practice, and effective applications. This book will contribute to the mix of small and big miracles that result from the combination of a great modality and great applied education.

The water has many healing benefits; in fact studies have shown that just sitting in a hot tub has measurable therapeutic value. Water is helpful even without wisdom, and due to the relative newness of the education of the industry, it requires much effort to collect the skills needed to be a great practitioner in water. It is even harder for the person with RA to find information that is helpful in healing from injury or disease. It has been common in the past to see those that work out in the water or those that teach them to do so with only surface knowledge. This book will help in changing this shortfall.

This book collects all the required pieces in plain, easily understood prose, providing a solid base for success. Both those who lead patients or clients with RA to better physical health and those with RA who wish to heal their body from dis-ease will benefit.

From the imparted experiential knowledge, the well-researched, up-to-date information, the clearly illustrated, well-described water exercise section, the putting it all together with knowledge from other disciplines, this book provides the foundation and the follow through needed to serve its audience very well. The audience for this book is very broad indeed. It serves the patient seeking wellness to the medical doctor and includes everyone in between, including but not limited to physical therapists, occupational therapists, massage therapists, recreation therapists, nurses, personal trainers, aquatic fitness instructors, medical exercise specialists, arthritis exercise instructors right down to the proactive clients that takes charge of their own health.

You will appreciate the clear descriptions of complex principles that make the point without bogging you down. The exercise list includes all the important exercises including some that I know are important for the client but are not often seen in other exercise protocols. No sifting through manuals to find what you need, it's all here in one efficient, very usable resource. If you teach others water exercise and therapy you will appreciate having the exercises in this book. If you suffer from RA and you seek background information on the disease to develop a health maintenance program, using this book will provide all that you need.

It is important that this book and others like it become increasingly more available and accessible to the mainstream markets, to those millions with arthritis, so that all can benefit from the knowledge and information contained within. Many lives have been improved, and even transformed by water, and this book is one of the ripples in the healing waters that will help continue the awareness and increase the success one can achieve in the journey to better health.

— Sheralee Beebe
Author of the Rheumatology Certification
for the Aquatic Therapy & Rehab Institute

Introduction

Water Exercises for Rheumatoid Arthritis explains how water exercise helps relieve the pains and restrictions caused by rheumatoid arthritis. The book will explain how exercises, in general, and water exercise, in particular, are excellent ways to maintain flexibility and mobility and reduce the pain and swelling caused by rheumatoid arthritis.

While the water exercises in this book are similar to the exercises in other books in this series, different conditions require different exercise programs and some modifications in the exercises themselves. The information in this book covers rheumatoid arthritis. Other books in this series look at osteoarthritis, fibromyalgia, and Parkinson's disease.

The book starts with a discussion of rheumatoid arthritis and how it affects your body. Next is how exercise helps you feel better, the basics of water exercise, and working with a companion. Finally, there are the exercises themselves. There are many different exercises here to give you a choice of programs that will be enjoyable and interesting. This book is written for people who have rheumatoid arthritis and their friends and family members. It can also be used by fitness instructors, personal trainers, physical therapists, and physicians to provide information to their clients or patients.

Benefits of Exercise

Let's start by looking at the benefits of exercise for a person with rheumatoid arthritis. Exercise can be defined as any physical activity

1

performed with planned, repetitious movement for the purpose of improving physical fitness. Exercise is an important part of the treatment process for people with rheumatoid arthritis. People with rheumatoid arthritis are just like anyone else in that they want to live active independent lives for as long as possible. The longer a person's bones, muscles, ligaments, and tendons are healthy, the longer a person will be able to climb stairs and get in and out of cars, chairs, and beds. They will also be able to take walks, garden, carry and lift children, groceries, books, and other items.

One of the unique benefits of exercise is ~~that~~ it increases a person's sense of body position (proprioception). A person who is fit has a better sense of space and alignment. When people maintain proprioception, they fall less. For example, very few twenty year olds stumble off of sidewalk curbs or steps, but plenty of sixty to seventy year olds do. Even when a younger person trips, proprioceptors in the joints send out warning signals that help the person reestablish balance and avoid a fall. Proprioceptive ability is lost without movement. Aerobic exercise helps to maintain proprioceptive abilities by keeping you aware of where your body is and what it is doing.

A big concern for people with rheumatoid arthritis is the use of the hands and fingers. Stiff, painful, swollen fingers make doorknobs, steering wheels, food packages, and medicine bottles a struggle. Keeping the hands and fingers as pain free and flexible as possible is just as important as maintaining the ability to walk.

People with rheumatoid arthritis, their families, and care providers should know the three basic reasons to include exercise as part of the overall treatment program. The first reason is that establishing an exercise program, with the aid of therapists and fitness professionals, helps people with rheumatoid arthritis and their families become more familiar and better educated about their condition. By being better informed, people with rheumatoid arthritis and their families will understand how rheumatoid arthritis affects their bodies, and how to compensate for their limitations.

The second reason is that exercise can slow the progress of rheumatoid arthritis as well as other diseases and ailments caused by a sedentary lifestyle. Often people with rheumatoid arthritis will experience pain and swelling of their joints and stop exercising. This leads to muscle atrophy, which leads to weakness and, ultimately, immobility. A lack of exercise can also lead to heart disease, cancer, depression, and obesity. Regular exercise keeps muscles supple and joints lubricated and flexible for a longer period of time. A daily exercise program prevents the vicious cycle of less activity leading to muscle loss, leading to less activity.

The third reason for people with rheumatoid arthritis to exercise is to improve their overall mental health. Exercise helps to increase muscle tone, strength, and flexibility and it improves your outlook on life. When you exercise with a companion or a group, you are interacting in a positive social manner, keeping your interpersonal interactions active. Exercise also releases endorphins that make you feel happier and more in control of your life.

Benefits of Water Exercise

Now let's look at why water is one of the best places to get your exercise. Fitness professionals and aquatic instructors know that water is an ideal element for several reasons. The key properties of the water are buoyancy, resistance force, hydrostatic pressure, and warmth.

Buoyancy counters the downward force of gravity that opposes the water's upward thrust. This decreases stress to the bones, joints, and muscles. Water envelops all of the submerged joints and limbs and acts as a cushion against jarring motions. The water's buoyancy helps to support your weight and helps to improve balance.

Resistance force is the water's ability to create resistance in all directions thus allowing the muscles to work in all directions. Water is a heavy fluid; therefore participants are constantly encountering resistance. The more exertion you use to move through the water, the more resistance you encounter. Resistance of the water can be four to 42 times greater than air. Walking three miles per hour in the water burns twice as many calories as walking three miles per hour on land.

Muscle conditioning in the water is different than using weight machines because weight machines stabilize the body except for the muscle group that is being exercised. In water the muscles are being worked on both sides of a joint in a balanced fashion. The abdominals act as the body's stabilizing force in the water instead of the body relying on stabilization from the weight machine.

As people with rheumatoid arthritis start to work in the water, they notice how much their abdominals are used to help them remain upright and balanced while performing various exercises. By maintaining balance and good upright posture, the chances of sustaining a fall-related injury decrease. It is important for people with rheumatoid arthritis to maintain confidence in their ability to keep a steady balance and good posture. If a person fears falling, fall-related injuries will increase and the ability to perform daily living activities will decrease. Since the muscles are worked in all directions, balance and strengthening occur at the same time.

Hydrostatic pressure is pressure from water that is exerted on the surface of an immersed body. Hydrostatic pressure increases resistance against the chest wall and forces the respiratory muscles to work more and become more efficient. It also helps to circulate the blood from the lower extremities back to the heart, which helps to lower blood pressure and improve the heart rate. Hydrostatic pressure helps reduce the swelling of inflamed joints and keeps the body's core stabilizers, or the torso, in an upright position.

Warmth is important because warm water soothes the joints and muscles of people with rheumatoid arthritis. Warm water helps muscles to relax, reduces rigidity, and allows the muscles to move more freely through a full range of motion.

1

Basics of Arthritis

Before we take a look at the specific condition of rheumatoid arthritis, let's take a look at all types of arthritis (including fibromyalgia). Arthritis is a medical term used to describe many different diseases that involve muscle aches, joint tenderness or swelling, inflammation, and disfigurement.

There are two major categories of arthritis: osteoarthritis and inflammatory arthritis. Osteoarthritis is the most common form of arthritis and is acquired through abnormal wear and tear of the cartilage caused by an injury or by carrying excessive weight. Inflammatory arthritis is a disease of the immune system and affects the lining of the joints more than the cartilage. Within the inflammatory category there are metabolic and immune system mediated types of arthritis. The most common metabolic type of arthritis is gout. Among the immune system mediated, the most common are rheumatoid arthritis and fibromyalgia.

Generally, arthritis occurs when the articular (connecting) cartilage fails to adequately protect the ends of the bones from trauma. The term "arthritis" is derived from the Greek words "arthron" meaning joint and "itis" meaning inflammation, thus arthritis means inflammation of a joint. Arthritis is widely used to refer to any condition that causes aches and pain in the joints, muscles, and connective tissues that surround the body's organs. Arthritis can range from very mild types with few symptoms to serious, crippling types.

Arthritis affects one in every three people in the U.S. and most families have a member or members who suffer from it. A 2001 study by the Centers for Disease Control and Prevention found that 70 million Americans, young and old, are affected. These numbers are 63% higher than the estimates of 1996 when it was thought 43 million people suffered from arthritis. This increase is associated with aging baby boomers, as well as better methods of gathering information.

Arthritis is found in people from all fifty states, but the

Table 1: Percentage of Adults Reporting Arthritis or Chronic Joint Symptoms

Lowest < 32.0%	Midrange 32.0% to 35.3%	Highest: 35.3%
Alaska	Arizona	Alabama
California	Delaware	Arkansas
Colorado	Florida	Idaho
Connecticut	Georgia	Indiana
District of Columbia	Illinois	Kentucky
Guam	Iowa	Maine
Hawaii	Kansas	Michigan
Maryland	Louisiana	Mississippi
Massachusetts	Minnesota	Missouri
Nebraska	Nevada	Montana
New Hampshire	New York	Ohio
New Jersey	North Carolina	Oklahoma
New Mexico	Rhode Island	Oregon
North Dakota	South Carolina	Pennsylvania
Puerto Rico	Vermont	Tennessee
South Dakota	Virginia	West Virginia
Texas	Washington	Wisconsin
U.S. Virgin Islands		
Utah		
Wyoming		

Source: CDC, Behavioral Risk Factor Surveillance System, 2001.

distribution is not even. The state with the lowest number of people with arthritis is Hawaii with 17.8% of adults having arthritis. West Virginia is the highest with 42%. Table 1 shows the prevalence of arthritis among the adult population in the United States.

There are many ways a person can develop arthritis. It can be brought on by injures, infections, genetic predisposition, wear and tear on the joints, defects in the immune system, and environmental factors. The symptoms of the disease become more noticeable in people over 45, but new studies indicate that arthritis actually starts when people are in their 30s or even as young as 20. By the time a person feels the first hint of arthritis, the degeneration of the bones and/or cartilage has already done damage to the joints. Gender makes a difference; women are twice as likely as men to have arthritis. While arthritis is most common in adults, more than 300,000 children are also affected.

Arthritis is a very costly disease. The lost wages and medical bills add up to $125 billion a year with 45 million lost workdays. Heart disease is the only disease that costs more. Arthritis is the most disabling disease in America and severely limits everyday activities for 7.9 million people. Arthritis affects 7.5% of all workers and is one of the most common reasons people leave the work force. People with arthritis average eight visits a year to their physicians compared to an average of four visits from people suffering from other chronic illnesses. Of the 70 million sufferers, six million are self-diagnosed and improperly self-treated. This allows mild symptoms of arthritis to become worse, as we will see later.

Before we look at the types of arthritis, we must examine what happens in a healthy joint. A joint is a location where two bones meet so that one bone can move in relation to the other bone. In the human body there are three kinds of joints: fibrous or fixed, cartilaginous or sliding, and synovial.

Fibrous joints, like the ones between the bones in the skull, are fixed and immobile and are not typically affected by arthritis.

Cartilaginous joints occur between the vertebra in the back and neck allowing the bones to slide along the cartilage. The cartilage between these joints may become worn and lead to osteoarthritis.

The rest of the joints are synovial joints. These joints are made of cartilage, joint space, capsule, synovium, and ligaments as shown in Figure 1. Cartilage is a smooth, white, slippery tissue that is attached to the bone and covers the bone ends. Joint space is the area between cartilages. Surrounding the cartilage and joint space is a soft, loose, fibrous capsule that permits movement of the joint. Within this bag like structure is a soft tissue, called the synovium. The synovium is a delicate, wet, smooth lining on the inner surface of the fibrous capsule that secretes a fluid called synovial fluid. This fluid acts as a lubricant and a waste disposal mechanism. The synovial fluid removes bacteria,

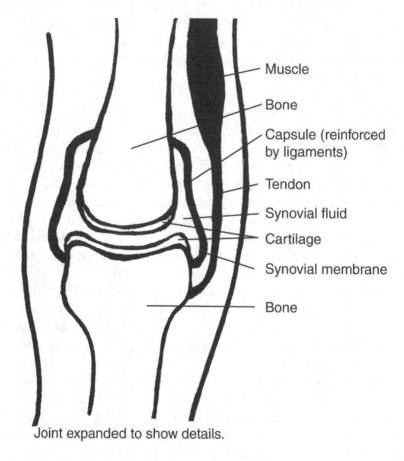

Joint expanded to show details.

Figure 1: A normal joint.

foreign tissue, and other waste material from the joint space; absorbs the waste into the synovial lining; and digests the material.

Ligaments are rope-like flexible structures that are located on the outside of the bone. Ligaments help to keep bones in proper alignment with one another. Collagen is a fibrous protein that is part of the structure of both bones and ligaments. When collagen is in the bone, it is calcified and stiff. Collagen in the ligament is not calcified and remains flexible. Different kinds of arthritis (and diseases related to arthritis) affect different parts of the joint.

Synovial joints are found in the hips, shoulders, knees, elbows, toes, neck, fingers, ankles, and wrists. Depending on the structure of the joint they may be called ellipsoidal, ball and socket, hinge, pivotal, and gliding.

Brief History of Arthritis

George Burns, a well-known comedian, was once asked if he had arthritis. He replied, "Have I had arthritis? I got it when it first came out!" George Burns was not too far off the mark. Arthritis has been around as long as humankind. Evaluations of the bones of Neanderthals from 40,000 to 100,000 years ago indicate that early humans suffered from arthritis. X-rays of mummies show that Egyptians suffered from arthritis. References to the disease are found in Greek and Roman literature. As early as 500 BC, the bark from the willow tree was used to relieve pain in the joints. Willow bark contains the naturally occurring compound salicylate. The synthesized version of willow bark later became the main ingredient in aspirin.

In 1819, Benjamin C. Brodie documented the effects of arthritis on the joints, tendons, and bursa. In 1858, A.B. Garrod coined the term "rheumatoid arthritis" and recognized that it was a separate disease with its own pathology. Around 1860, a French neurologist, Guillanme Benjamin Arman Duchenne, used electric current from a battery to ease the pain of his patients with chronic rheumatism. Although Dr. Duchenne was trying to practice good medicine, the use of electricity in the form of gadgets and magnets soon became a medium used by charlatans.

About the same time, another French doctor, Jean Martin Charcot, was experimenting with hydrotherapy to treat joint pain and inflammation. Dr. Charcot used warm circulating water on his patients. Dr. Charcot is considered the father of the study of neurology. In 1867 Dr. Charcot went a little further than Garrod and recognized that gout, rheumatic fever, osteoarthritis, and rheumatoid arthritis were all separate conditions. Augustine Jacob Landre-Beauvais of France made the first clinical description of rheumatoid arthritis in 1880.

By 1897, aspirin was being used to treat arthritis pain and inflammation. Aspirin was the first member of a new class of medicines called nonsteroidal anti-inflammatory drugs (NSAIDs). NSAIDs work by blocking the enzyme cyclooxygenase or COX, which produces prostaglandins. Prostaglandins are a group of hormone-like substances produced from amino acids in the tissue that are responsible for a wide range of physiological functions such as nerve transmission, metabolism, and smooth muscle activity. Some prostaglandins help to keep the stomach lining healthy, regulate blood pressure, regulate blood flow to the kidneys, and enable the blood to clot. However, other prostaglandins cause fever, pain, and inflammation in joints and muscles. Aspirin blocks the prostaglandins that cause fever, pain, and inflammation, but at the same time aspirin also blocks the prostaglandins that protect the stomach lining.

In 1929 another class of medicines was developed called disease-modifying antirheumatic drugs (DMARDs). DMARDs are derived from gold salts and used to relieve the pain of rheumatoid arthritis. Some DMARDs started out as medications for other aliments such as cancer and malaria. Often, the people who had these illnesses also had arthritis. It became apparent that the medications helped not only the primary disease, but also the symptoms of rheumatoid arthritis. For example, methotrexate was developed to treat cancer; cyclosporine is used to stop the body from rejecting transplanted organs; and hydroxychloroquine is a drug used to treat malaria. Yet they all help with symptoms of rheumatoid arthritis. The full impact of NSAIDs and DMARDs will be addressed in the chapter on safety.

Rheumatoid Arthritis

Rheumatoid arthritis is an autoimmune disease. Symptoms differ from person to person but the most common symptoms of rheumatoid arthritis are inflamed joints, pain, stiffness of the joints, and a feeling of the joints being on fire. It occurs because the body's own immune system treats organs and tissues as foreign, hostile invaders and attacks them.

Rheumatoid arthritis is a chronic disease that has periods of flare-ups and remission. The process of the body's immune system malfunctioning and attacking healthy tissue has three major attributes: Blood vessels dilate and increase the blood flow to the area. White blood cells infiltrate the area to fight the perceived infection. Fluid in the blood leaks into the tissues causing edema or swelling. This results in four typical symptoms: swelling, redness, warmth, and pain. The white blood cells break down the bone and collagen as if the bone and collagen were the enemy.

Rheumatoid arthritis can affect up to 15-20 joints at a time. When only one joint is involved, it is called monoarticular rheumatoid arthritis. When it affects more than one joint, it is called polyarticular rheumatoid arthritis. Rheumatoid arthritis can involve other tissues such as the lungs, spleen, skin, and even the heart. However the majority of the problems involve joint damage and pain.

Rheumatic diseases, including rheumatoid arthritis, have been around for a long time. Descriptions have been found in the writings of the ancient Greek physician, Hippocrates. In North America, skeletal remains from 3000 years ago show evidence of rheumatoid arthritis lesions. In the 1st century AD in Europe, physicians thought the disease was caused by blockages in the "humors" that flowed through the body. Humors in medieval times referred to the body's fluids. They reasoned that the pain and swelling were caused by the humors getting blocked by the joints when they bent. The name rheumatoid arthritis comes from the word "rheuma" which means a "substance that flows."

The American College of Rheumatology (ACR) first developed criteria to diagnose rheumatoid arthritis in 1958 and revised the criteria in 1987. According to the ACR, if a person displays four of these seven conditions they have rheumatoid arthritis:

- morning stiffness that occurs within the joint and other surrounding joints and lasts at least an hour before subsiding
- three or more joint areas experiencing soft-tissue swelling
- abnormal amounts of rheumatoid factor
- rheumatoid nodules
- arthritis of hand joints
- symmetric arthritis
- radiographic changes.

Today, rheumatoid arthritis affects about one percent of the adult population or 5.8 million people worldwide and 2.1 million Americans. The specific cause is unknown, however genetics and

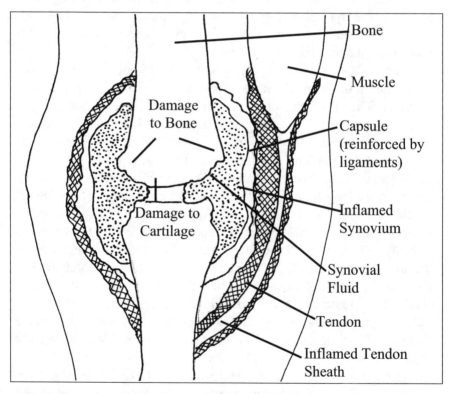

Figure 2: A joint with rheumatoid arthritis.

smoking seem to predispose some people to a higher risk. Rikard Holmdahl, a professor at Sweden's Lund University and his colleges were able to locate a gene they believe is responsible for rheumatoid arthritis in rats. The researchers were able to block the onset of arthritis in the rats through this gene but it will be years before this kind of medicine will be available for humans.

The primary target of rheumatoid arthritis is the synovium. (See Figure 2.) When it is healthy, the synovium is velvety and smooth. With rheumatoid arthritis, the synovium becomes inflamed, rough, granulated, and swollen. A diseased synovium viewed under a microscope shows the presence of lymphocytes, plasma cells, and macrophages, which are elements of the body's immune system. The presence of these cells indicates that rheumatoid arthritis may be a virus-initiated disease. There is speculation that synovial tissue contains an antigen (a foreign substance). Scientists think that one of the antigens present may actually be a virus. The body's attempt to reject the virus is what causes the pain and swelling, resulting in the destruction of the synovial layer.

The antigen/virus theory is supported by the presence of antibody production. Plasma cells produce antibodies called "rheumatoid factor" to fight the virus. This is similar to the method our bodies use to fight diseases after we have been given a vaccine. Since a virus has never been found in rheumatoid arthritis tissue, scientists are not sure what causes the body to produce rheumatoid factor. However, the virus theory has the most support for now. A similar theory with less support is that mycobacteria (rod-shaped bacteria) may be present in the tissues of the joint. Usually the immune system can't detect these. Under certain circumstances, especially stress, the immune system notices mycobacteria and tries to destroy them, destroying the joint tissues as well.

When the immune system attacks the synovium, the white blood cells replace the synovium with cells called pannus, a destructive mass of blood vessels and other cells. Part of the stiffness from rheumatoid arthritis is caused because pannus is thicker than synovium and does not allow nutrients to get through to the joint. Normal, healthy synovium is only two to three cell layers thick, but pannus is hundreds of cell layers thick. With healthy synovium (which is thin, slippery, and porous) vitamins, glucose, amino acids, fats, and oxygen get through to nourish the joint. The thicker, less porous layer of pannus does not allow for the nourishment of the joint so the joint becomes malnourished and incapable of repairing itself.

In addition to problems at the joints, rheumatoid arthritis causes changes affecting the whole body. The immune response discussed above increases the metabolic rate by about 20%. Increased metabolism places greater demands on the body for food. In addition, the immune system secretes cytokines. These create chemical signals that change the fuel mix from fat and carbohydrates to mostly protein and little fat. The body often lacks sources for protein in this mix so it will break down muscle tissue in order to provide itself with protein, which causes the muscles to deteriorate.

In a healthy person, there is a 20% decrease of muscle mass from the age of 20 to the age of 70. People in their 70s who have rheumatoid arthritis will lose 33% of their muscle mass and a decrease of 40% muscle mass can be fatal.

Eating more protein will not necessarily provide the muscles with more protein. If a person eats protein, the immune system will take what it needs and the excess will be stored as fat. Even with a higher metabolism, people with rheumatoid arthritis store fat more easily then those who do not have rheumatoid arthritis because of the change in their fuel mix.

When people have rheumatoid arthritis, weight is not a good measure of the amount of body fat. The metabolic changes mean the body's muscle to fat ratio is lower. So even if people with rheumatoid arthritis are not overweight, they may still have poor muscle tone and too much fat. This cycle causes fatigue, physical weakness, reduced activity, and more muscle loss. The result is a higher risk for stroke and heart disease. The risk of stroke, heart disease, and muscle deterioration are some of the reasons why the mortality rate for people with rheumatoid arthritis is two to five times greater than the general population.

It is possible to improve the odds. Making choices to reduce stress, improve eating, and increasing the amount of healthy exercise will go a long way toward reducing the problems associated with rheumatoid arthritis.

2

Exercise with Arthritis

The pain of arthritis causes many people to stop exercising and leaves them vulnerable to all of the health risks associated with a sedentary lifestyle, such as heart disease, high blood pressure, obesity, cancer, and diabetes.

Everyone knows that exercise is an important part of a healthy lifestyle. What might be less obvious is rather than making arthritis worse, exercise actually helps you get better. For example, regular exercise helps reduce the pain and stiffness of osteoarthritis and can slow the progression of osteoporosis (weakening of the bones). In fact, exercise can increase bone density as much as two to eight percent a year.

Exercise also helps to maintain proper weight. This is important because excess weight can accelerate the onset of arthritis, especially osteoarthritis and rheumatoid arthritis. Women who are overweight are four times more likely and men who are overweight are five times more likely to have osteoarthritis of the knee. Being only 10 pounds overweight can increase the pressure on the knees by 30 to 60 pounds with each step. The Framingham Knee Osteoarthritis Study showed the relationship between weight loss and arthritis. It concluded that if a person lost an average of 10 pounds over a 10-year period the risk of osteoarthritis of the knee was cut by 50%.

Two-thirds of the people who have rheumatoid arthritis experience pain and limited movement. A smaller but significant number of people with arthritis are unable to perform daily activities because of pain and movement limitations. Exercise helps decrease the pain and increase movement. The longer you are able to maintain your ability to remain active, the longer you will be independent. All of these facts emphasize that exercise is an important part of an overall health plan for a person who has arthritis.

Types of Exercise

The types of exercises that are best for a person with arthritis depends on the type of arthritis you have, the joints that are affected, and the severity of the disease. The general benefits of exercise for most types of arthritis include: increased flexibility, improved cardiovascular endurance and muscle strength, reduced joint pain and stiffness, increased bone mass, improved sleep, less fatigue, weight loss, stronger bones, and healthier cartilage.

There are three types of exercises that are helpful for all people with arthritis. They are range-of-motion (ROM) and stretching exercises, strengthening exercises, and endurance exercises.

Range-of-Motion and Stretching Exercises

ROM exercises reduce stiffness, improve flexibility, help to flush out waste products from the joints, and restore the synovial fluid that keeps joints lubricated. ROM exercises can be done daily and involve moving the joints in certain directions normally and frequently. These exercises, along with stretching exercises, are especially beneficial for people who have rheumatoid arthritis.

There are three types of ROM exercises: passive, active assistive, and active. Passive ROM occurs when another person performs movement on you. It is used when you need help accomplishing an exercise because you cannot move effectively on your own. An example would be allowing a physical therapist to move your arm through a series of motions. When the therapist or fitness trainer uses passive ROM to move your limb you are using little or no muscle strength to accomplish the motion. Passive ROM does not strengthen a muscle but keeps the muscles, ligaments, and joints lubricated and flexible.

Active-assistive ROM occurs when the participant performing the ROM exercise is assisted by another person or when the participant performs the exercise with the help of equipment or special exercise techniques. An example of active-assistive ROM using equipment would be for you to use an exercise machine that incorporates pulleys or counterbalance weights. An example of active-assistive ROM using an exercise technique would be engaging in water exercises where the buoyancy of the water assists you with the motion. With active-assistive ROM, you provide some or most of the muscle strength required while the exercise equipment or exercise technique provides the rest of the energy needed.

Active ROM occurs when you perform the exercises unassisted using your own strength to perform all of the exercise. Equipment or stretching techniques can also be incorporated. With active ROM, equipment is used to challenge your strength level by adding resistance. An exercise technique such as water exercise can be used to add resistance through the properties of drag and water resistance.

Strength Exercises

Strength exercises strengthen the muscles, bones, and joints. They include isometric exercises where the muscles are contracted but the joints are not moved and isotonic exercises where the joints are moved to strengthen the muscles. Strong muscles help to support the joints.

An example of an isometric exercise would be putting the hands together and pushing on the palms. This strengthens the muscles of the arms by forcing them to remain contracted for an extended period of time. An example of an isotonic exercise would be leg extension. The knee joint is used as a lever to help lift the lower leg. The movement strengthens the quadriceps muscle, which is located in the front of the thigh. When joints are stronger and more stable, a person is able to move about with more ease and less pain. Isometric exercises are especially beneficial for helping to strengthen joints that are impaired. Strengthening exercises should be done every other day unless severe pain or swelling develops.

When muscles are exercised, they work in opposing but synchronized pairs. As a muscle flexes or shortens, the opposing muscle extends or lengthens. The muscles performing the actual work are called agonists. As agonist muscles contract, the opposing muscles, called antagonists, relax to allow the movement to continue. In the return move, the roles of the muscles are reversed. Figure 3 shows

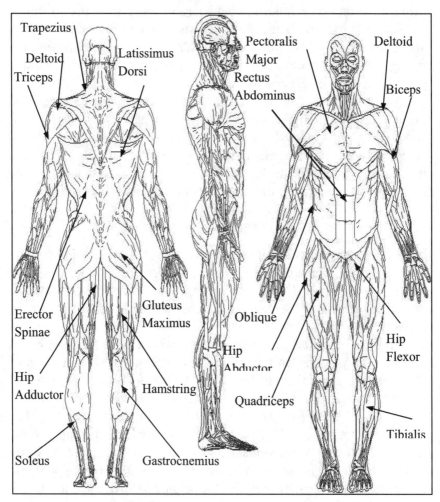

Figure 3: Muscle diagram

some important muscle groups. Examples of opposing muscle groups
are

- quadriceps/hamstrings
- biceps/triceps
- hip adductors/abductors
- pectoralis major/trapezius and latissimus dorsi
- hip flexor/gluteus
- gastrocnemius/tibialis
- erector spinae/rectus abdominis.

All muscle pairs have an ideal ratio of strength. When the ratio is
out of balance, possibly due to training only one of the muscles in a
pair, the body works inefficiently and the muscle pair puts stress on
the joint. A person with arthritis is at more risk for joint and muscle
injury.

Endurance Exercises

Endurance exercises improve stamina and sleep, strengthen the
heart, control weight, and give you a sense of well being. These
exercises bring the heart rate up to 65-85% of the maximum heart rate
for an extended period of time strengthening the heart and lungs so
they perform at their peak efficiency. Table 2 shows target heart rates
as a function of age for a person in good health and normal condition.
It is strongly recommend, especially if you are on any heart
medication, that you consult your doctor about your heart rate before
doing endurance exercises.

Some of the preferred endurance exercises are walking, biking,
swimming, and water exercises. These particular exercises, especially
water exercises, put less strain and pressure on the joints than
running, high impact aerobics, racquetball, and tennis. Water helps to
support the body allowing the joints to move through their full range
of motion. Endurance exercises that are performed in the water are
especially beneficial for people who have rheumatoid arthritis
because the buoyancy of the water helps keep weight and pressure off
of the hips, knees, and spine.

Endurance exercises should be done at least three times a week
for at least 20 to 30 minutes unless there is severe joint pain. If it is

not convenient to exercise 20 to 30 minutes continuously, the session can be broken down into 10 to 15 minute sessions two to three times during the day.

Interval Training

Interval training can be part of an endurance and strength training program. It involves quick spurts of rapid movement or very intense movement incorporated into an aerobic program. The rapid movements increase the energy requirements of the muscles beyond the aerobic threshold into the anaerobic zone. When intervals are done for 30 to 60 seconds, they increase the heart rate momentarily. (Get a doctors approval before trying it.) When a person trains using an alternating pattern of intense intervals and aerobic recovery intervals, they are training the heart to respond to specific needs of the body.

Table 2: Target Heart Rate Training Zones

Age	50% Zone	75% Zone	Max. Rate
20	100	150	200
25	98	146	195
30	95	142	190
35	93	138	185
40	90	135	180
45	88	131	175
50	85	127	170
55	83	123	165
60	80	120	160
65	78	116	155
70	75	113	150

Exercise and Rheumatoid Arthritis

With rheumatoid arthritis the major goals of an exercise program are to maintain a healthy synovial fluid system in the joints, reduce pain and swelling especially after a period of inactivity or sleep, and alleviate fatigue. Increasing general fitness and reducing excess weight should be part of any exercise program. Exercises that strengthen the muscles and improve the movement of the joints are an important goal.

For people with rheumatoid arthritis, endurance exercises are especially important. These exercises reduce the level of fatigue, maintain the level of synovial fluid in the joint capsule and help to maintain the circulatory and lymph systems in the joint and for the whole body, allowing the joint to repair itself to some degree.

Strength exercises help to keep the bones and muscles strong and dense alleviating the swelling and soreness associated with rheumatoid arthritis. Stronger muscles support the joints making them more stable. After exercising regularly, people with rheumatoid arthritis notice they are not as sore and stiff upon waking in the morning and have fewer episodes of stiffness during the day. Fatigue is reduced by strength exercises because the exercises build stronger muscles.

Range of motion exercises increase the degree of movement within the joints and muscles and improve the flow of the synovial fluids in the joint. The pressure from gentle movement helps the swollen tissues release excess fluid, which reduces stiffness.

Endurance and strength exercises increase the body's muscle to fat ratio. Muscle tone is increased and excess fat is reduced increasing general health and causing a reduction in the amount of fatigue and pain experienced.

For a long time, people with rheumatoid arthritis have been cautioned against engaging in intense exercise and have been advised to participate in more conservative activities. Intense exercises include biking, jogging, or even walking. Conservative activities are stretching and isometric strengthening exercises. Dr. C.H.M. Van den Ende of the University Hospital in Leiden, The Netherlands, believes conservative exercise regimes do not provide enough conditioning to be adequately effective for people with rheumatoid arthritis. He believes people with arthritis who do not have an adequate exercise program make their arthritis worse by gaining weight through inactivity placing their joints at more risk for pain.

Dr. Van den Ende conducted a study involving 64 people with rheumatoid arthritis who had the disease for an average of eight years. Groups were chosen to participate in either an intensive exercise regimen or a conservative exercise program. The intensive exercise program consisted of resistance training five times a week and aerobic training three times a week plus range of motion exercises and isometric exercises. The intensive exercise program was reduced during flare-ups. The conservative program consisted of only range of motion exercises and isometric exercises. During the 24-week study the participants were evaluated for progression of the disease, pain, functional ability, and strength.

The results showed that both groups improved in all areas, but the group that engaged in the intensive exercise program showed greater improvement in functional ability and muscle strength. The researchers concluded that intensive exercise was more effective in improving muscle strength than more cautious or conservative exercise programs.

Just a personal note: I exercise intensely and use a personal trainer on occasion. My trainer is a delightful young woman who is fit, active, and knowledgeable and has rheumatoid arthritis. Rheumatoid arthritis is not slowing her down, nor should it slow anyone else down.

Let's look at some of the other research examining exercise and rheumatoid arthritis.

In a study conducted at Tufts, a group of people with rheumatoid arthritis engaged in a strength-training program using exercise machines twice a week for 45 minutes. The people worked their legs, chest, back, and abdominal muscles. After three months, the muscle strength in those areas increased by 54% to 75%. Balance improved and participants were able to walk faster and more easily and reported less joint pain and fatigue.

In a study reported in the *Annals of the Rheumatic Diseases*, 15 people with rheumatoid arthritis were studied for a period of two to three years. Half of the people did physical exercise and the other half did not. Those who did not exercise had a four percent loss of bone mass from their outer forearm. Physical activity maintains bone mass and helps to prevent fractures.

Overall we can see that exercise will help a person with rheumatoid arthritis. Endurance and strength-building exercises are especially important for improving functional ability and strength. Adding range of motion exercises improves joint mobility. All reduce the pain and swelling. Again, it is important to remember that exercise is usually a good idea, but exercising intensely during a flare-up of rheumatoid arthritis should be avoided.

Water Exercise and Arthritis

The use of water therapy for arthritis is one of the oldest methods of rehabilitation and dates back to the Roman Empire. At that time, water therapy consisted of sitting in hot or cold whirlpool baths. Today, water therapy in the form of water exercise is ideal for people who have rheumatoid arthritis. Before embarking on a water exercise program, you should consult your doctor. Initially, it would be wise to train with a fitness professional or a physical therapist in order to make sure the exercise program is the best one for you. Begin slowly and progress gradually. Try to include all three basic types of exercise in a water exercise program: ROM, strength, and endurance. Warm-up and cool down with each session. Before exercising, try using heat by sitting in a whirlpool or sauna to help warm up the joints. Use cold packs after exercise to keep swelling down. If exercise becomes painful and unpleasant, stop and consult your physician. Exercise is most beneficial when it is a regular part of an established routine.

When you are in the water, your body will have a tendency to float. Grounding movements such as walking in the water are movements that help the body resist the urge to float. Grounding movements are generally done in an upright position.

The density of water allows you to work in a wide variety of planes. These are the vertical or sagittal, the frontal or coronal, and the transverse or horizontal plane. The vertical plane divides the body into right and left halves, the frontal plane divides the body into front and back halves, and horizontal plane divides the body into upper and lower halves. There are common movements done in each of these planes. In the vertical plane, adduction (moving toward the midline) and abduction (moving away from the midline) are common movements. In the frontal plane a typical movement would involve flexion and extension. In the horizontal plane, medial and lateral rotation would be typical movements. Working in the water allows the body to move easily in multiple planes. (See Figure 4.)

There are six types of water activities that improve physical fitness.

- The first activity emphasizes range of motion. The buoyancy of water facilitates a pain-free range of motion.
- The second type of activity is walking or jogging slowly in the water and emphasizes proper gait patterns.
- The third type of activity focuses on vigorous exercises that strengthen the muscles and increase muscular endurance.
- The fourth uses the properties of the water to offer greater resistance in all of the planes and increases the use of functional

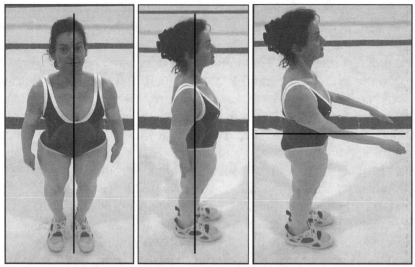

Figure 4: Vertical, Frontal, and Horizontal Planes

proprioceptive neuromuscular facilitation patterns.
- The fifth activity involves cardiovascular fitness such as running and jogging.
- The final activity is swimming. Swimming combines strength training and cardiovascular training into one activity.

Studies have shown that water exercises have positive effects on arthritis. In one study, 87 people who had arthritis and participated in water aerobic classes were compared to 174 people with arthritis who were in a rheumatic disease clinic. The groups were matched for age, sex, and type of arthritis. For participants who did not engage in water exercise, pain and disability were 7% higher and depression was 3% higher.

People with rheumatoid arthritis are at risk for low cardiovascular ability and low muscle strength. Performing low-impact exercises in a warm pool can increase isometric, isokinetic, and aerobic abilities. Dr. Peter J. Maddison, a rheumatologist and professor at the University of Bath in England, did a study involving 140 people with arthritis. Some of the participants exercised on dry land, some did progressive-relaxation exercises, some just sat in warm water, while the rest exercised in the warm water. The water exercises included water walking and special ROM exercises. All of the participants were supervised by a physical therapist. After four weeks the results showed that people in the hydrotherapy group saw the greatest improvements in their physical, emotional, and psychological state. Physically, the people who engaged in water therapy found walking easier, and other activities of daily living were easier because their joints were not so stiff. All of the participants who were in warm water, whether doing exercise or not, noticed a reduction in the swelling of their joints.

In a study reported in the May 2000 issue of Physical Therapy, people with arthritis were evaluated to see what results water exercises had on their quality of life, their balance, and their fear of falling due to impaired balance. The 21 participants were aged 60-85, of both genders and had either osteoarthritis or rheumatoid arthritis. The study lasted six weeks. The results of the study showed that water exercises contributed to better physical functioning and positive social interaction.

In another study involving people with rheumatoid arthritis, two groups were compared. One group exercised on a stationary bicycle and the other group did water running in a pool using a flotation device like a jogging belt or a water vest. The study wanted to evaluate whether water exercise could provide participants with the same training levels as a stationary bicycle (as set by the American College of Sports Medicine).

Eight women with adult-onset rheumatoid arthritis participated in the study. The women were 30 to 40 years of age and, despite having arthritis, were active and healthy. Some of the women rode the stationary bicycle reaching 60% of their maximum heart rate. The other women exercised in the water and achieved comparable heart rates.

The results of the study showed the participants were able to reach and maintain an aerobic level of training both on the bicycle and in the water. Neither method of exercise exacerbated the level of pain in the joints or muscles. Water, however, proved to be a better choice for people who had limited mobility and limited ROM in their lower extremities. The water cushioned their joints and helped them to maintain their balance.

The Arthritis Foundation has sponsored formal water exercise programs for people with arthritis and water exercise is widely accepted and valued by patients and professionals. However, little is known about the severity of arthritis in those who attend these programs and whether the programs reach those with significant musculoskeletal problems. In the state of Kansas, a group of 87 participants in water exercise programs and 174 patients attending a rheumatic disease clinic were studied by matching for type of arthritis, age, and sex. The mean age of the subjects was 66 years old and 82% were women. The clinic group, which did not engage in water exercise, showed significantly more pain, functional impairment, and global impact of the disease than the water exercise group. This difference was measured with the Health Assessment Questionnaire. Anxiety and depression, as measured by two subscales of the Arthritis Impact Measurement Scale, were increased for the clinic group. Program members with rheumatoid arthritis who engaged in water exercises had significantly higher grip strength and reported less global disease severity than the clinic group.

In another study, people with rheumatoid arthritis, along with a control group, assessed the effects of warm water exercises on the strength of the lower extremities. After engaging in a water program twice a week for eight weeks, the subjects had increased the strength of their quadriceps by 38% after performing isometric exercises and 16% after performing isokinetic exercises. There was also an increase in aerobic capacity. After participating in the water program, the subjects noticed an increased ability to perform activities of daily living and enjoyed more freedom of movement.

3

Safety

There are a number of safety concerns for you to consider when planning a water exercise program. These points are exercise safety, pool temperature, pool access, transportation, building access, clothing, and medications. A lot of the information in this chapter deals with common sense ideas that you are probably doing already. It is just a good idea to go through the list to make sure that the exercise program is as enjoyable and successful as possible.

Exercise Safety

Dr. Neil Gordon, director of exercise physiology at the Cooper Institute for Aerobics Research in Dallas, Texas has nine safety points people with rheumatoid arthritis need to consider before undertaking an exercise program:

- You should obtain a medical evaluation of your condition and continue to have regular medical evaluations.
- You should assess whether a medically supervised program is needed.
- You should know the warning signs of cardiac complications.
- You should make safety the first priority in your exercise program.
- You should engage in exercise that is not stressful or painful to

29

the joints.
- You should educate yourself on rheumatoid arthritis, the extent of joint inflammation and pain, and how exercise affects your condition.
- You should not ignore negative changes in functional ability, pain, or inflammation.
- You should not participate in passive forms of exercise without the guidance of a qualified professional.
- If you are taking anti-inflammatory medications, you should exercise when the medications are working at their peak.

Safety in the Water

When working out in the water it is important to work within your limitations. If you have a slight to mild case of arthritis, you will be able to exercise more vigorously than if you have more severe and limiting arthritis.

The exercises presented *Water Exercises for Rheumatoid Arthritis* offer a wide variety of choices for people at various levels of fitness and flexibility. You may not be able to do all of the exercises in the book, especially when you are just starting an exercise program. Please choose exercises that are fun and challenging to you at your level of fitness and based on the progression of your disease. Do not persist if the exercises become painful.

Range of motion and especially rotational movements of the hips, wrists, and shoulders will vary depending on the location and severity of your arthritis. Everyone with rheumatoid arthritis has individual needs from an exercise program. The wide variety of exercises that are in the book allow you to make choices to suit your particular condition. Pay attention to your own body to decide which exercises to do when designing a program.

Arthritis in the shoulders, hips, and wrists would suggest doing rotation exercises very carefully and slowly. Arthritis in the shoulders will not prevent a person from doing biceps strength training exercises or triceps strength training exercises as long as the upper arm is kept close to the body. Arthritis in the back means you should do rotation exercises at the waist very carefully to avoid hyperextension of the spine. Other exercises that need to be done slowly and carefully if there is arthritis in the back are tuck exercises that involve side to side or up and down movements. If you have arthritis in the back, you may wish to do tuck exercises in the supine position allowing the water to provide maximum cushioning. If you have arthritis in the hips, exercises involving hip movements in rotation, lateral movements, and movements front to back need to be executed slowly and carefully.

Range of motion will vary from person to person depending on the severity and stiffness inherent with the problems of arthritis. In fact, it will vary from day to day. The good news is that with continued effort and monitoring, range of motion will improve over time.

Another related issue is using the depth of the water appropriately. Since these are water exercises, I'm sure you understand that you almost always need to be in water deep enough for the part being exercised to be under the water. What might not be as clear is the advantage of using particular depths of water. For example, deep-water exercises with a jogging belt will let you do vigorous exercises while the water cushions sore and painful joints from the shoulders on down. Chest deep water offers the opportunity to work both the joints of the upper and lower body while still providing a cushioning effect. Water that is waist deep will cushion the joints of the lower body. If you are moving through the water, lower water levels will require less effort because there is less resistance and drag.

Here are some other things to consider regarding safety in the water.

Before you enter the pool you should be aware of the pool exits and the depth of the water in the different parts of the pool. Knowing where the exit steps or ramps are allows you to exercise an appropriate distance from the stairs/ramps so entry and exit is smooth and comfortable. Knowing where the depth changes allows you to transition from exercises in waist-deep water to exercises in chest-deep water easily.

It is best to stay close to the edge of the pool in case balance becomes an issue or if your knees and hips have limited range of motion. If you have arthritis primarily in the lower body, it may be necessary to hold on to the edge of the pool to stabilize yourself. Another alternative is to have a companion in the water with you to offer support. Other alternatives for people with severe arthritis are to use a waterproof cane with four prongs at the bottom or even a walker.

Unless you have a mild case with only a few joints affected and are an excellent swimmer, you probably should not work out in the water alone. Even if you are in good enough condition to do lap swimming, it is advisable that the facility's management and family members know where you are. Working with a trainer or a companion offers not only physical support, but also social and emotional interaction that makes exercising more enjoyable. Having another person in the water can also offer comfort and support for people who enjoy working out in the water but do not know how to swim. Another advantage is that the companion can watch for signs of excessive exertion and fatigue and help you exit the pool and return to the locker room if you overdo it a little.

Most of all, working out in the water requires using common sense so the experience is fun and productive for you and your companion. One common mistake is to exercise without eating and drinking enough. If exercising in the morning is the best time for you, be sure to have an adequate breakfast that is healthy and nutritious. As an instructor of many years, I have had people complain of lightheadedness in the middle of a class only to find out that they have not had anything to eat in the last 12 hours. Take care of yourself. I remember having a man collapse on the locker room floor because he worked out that morning on a totally empty stomach, ran out of energy, and had a hypoglycemic (low blood sugar) reaction that caused him to pass out. Eat and drink enough before you exercise, I don't ever want to be scared like that again.

If you take medications that have side effects, know what they are and whether they pose any risks such as drowsiness, hyperactivity, constipation, diarrhea, or nausea. Any one of these complications may take your focus away from the exercises and make the experience unpleasant and unproductive. Side effects from medications may become exaggerated from the heat when using the whirlpool, steam room, or dry sauna. This is not to say you shouldn't exercise, of course. Just try to find the best time for exercise in your medication schedule.

The goal of exercise is to get healthier and feel better. Being safe and comfortable in the water is a big part of that. So be prepared to exercise, stay safe in the pool, enter and exit the pool carefully, and then you will be prepared to enjoy the rest of your day.

Pool Temperature

Pool temperature is an important factor for people with rheumatoid arthritis. Cool water temperatures will cause muscles to contract and tighten. This makes people with rheumatoid arthritis feel stiff and makes putting the muscles through a full range of motion difficult and painful. Most therapeutic pools are kept at 93-95°F although the Arthritis Foundation recommends a temperature from 83-90°F with the air temperature the same as the water temperature or slightly higher. When the water temperature is at the lower end of the recommended scale, more vigorous exercises can be performed. At high temperatures slower stretching-type exercises are better. Working vigorously in water at the high end of the temperature range can cause you to become overheated and prematurely exhausted.

Pool Access

Pool access is another consideration. People with arthritis, fibromyalgia, and other disabilities represent 14% of the population that uses pools. In choosing a place to exercise pay attention to how safe and easy it is to enter and exit the pool. In 1996, the National Center on Accessibility devised the pool accessibility guidelines. These are

- There should be at least one means of accessible water entry/exit.
- Swimming pools with more than 300 linear feet of pool edge

should have at least two accessible water entry/exits.

- If only one entry/exit exists, it should be a wet ramp, zero-depth entry, or a lift chair.
- If a second entry/exit exists, it should be transfer steps, moveable floor, ramp, lift chair, or zero-depth entry.
- Ramps, lifts, and zero-depth entry should be used as only one means of entry/exit when other access is available.
- Both ends and sides of the pool should be served if there are two accessible entry/exits provided.

People with disabilities have five methods of safely entering a pool besides using ordinary stairs. These are zero-depth entry, lift chairs, transfer walls and steps, dry ramps, and moveable floors. People with disabilities prefer the zero-depth entry or lifts and ramps to moveable floors. Here is a look at each of these.

Zero-Depth Entry (ZDE) (Figure 5)

The zero-depth entry is the most widely used and preferred method of entry by both the general and disabled population. ZDE

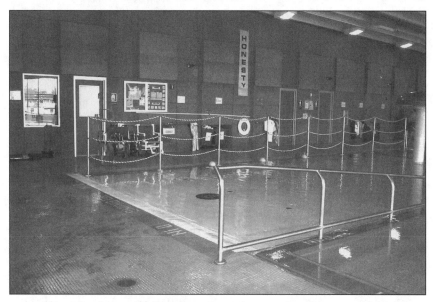

Figure 5: Zero-depth entry.

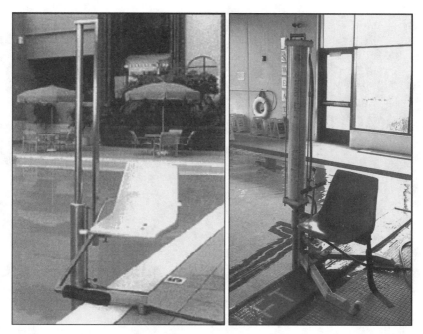

Figure 6: Examples of lift chairs

was originally designed to mimic an ocean beachfront and is used in wave pools at water parks. Access starts at a zero-depth and slopes gradually to the bottom of the pool. This method of pool entry is also ideal for anyone using an aquatic wheel chair.

Lifts (Figure 6)

Lifts are waterproof chairs or swings that are anchored on the side of the pool. The chair swings out over the water and then can be lowered to transfer you from the ledge to the water. The lifts are operated with an electric motor, water pressure, or a hand crank. They can also be used to transfer a person from a wheel chair in and out of the pool.

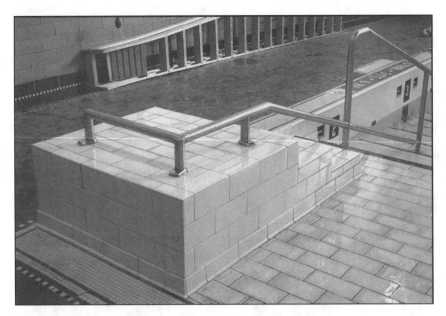

Figure 7: Transfer steps with steps into the water

Transfer Steps (Figure 7)

Transfer steps are portable or permanent raised tiers that are used for semi-recessed pools. Transfer steps allow a person to transfer from a wheelchair or crutches into the pool by holding the rails and sliding sideways onto the top tier and working themselves down the steps into the water.

Ramps (Figure 8)

Ramps are a modification of ZDE and are the most efficient and the easiest entry/exit system. Ramps are placed on the wall of the pool allowing a person to slide gradually into the water. They require less space and can be put alongside an in-ground pool. Some ramps are portable while others are permanently built into the side wall of the pool.

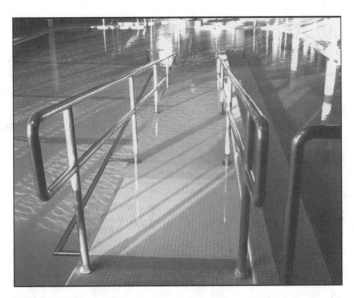

Figure 8: Ramp

Moveable Floors (Figure 9)

Moveable floors move up and down using a hinged trailing ramp, a vertical elevator, or a rolling bulkhead. They allow the pool to be entered at zero-depth and then slope down to the pool bottom. Moveable floors can cover part of the pool or the entire pool surface. A fully raised floor helps pools retain heat, prevents evaporation, and offers security from unauthorized entry. Of all of the entry/exit methods, the moveable floor is the most expensive and least favorite.

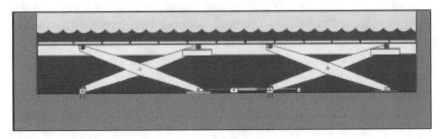

Figure 9: Diagram of how a moveable floor operates.

Facility Access

When choosing a facility with a pool, you need to consider how easy it is to access the facility, the equipment, and the pool. If you are going to start an exercise program, you need to be able to get to a health club or community facility that has an accessible building entrance, pool, and equipment.

Transportation

Transportation and parking are big considerations. If you do not drive, then you may need to use public transportation or rely on family members or friends. If family members and friends are the means of transportation, they will need to drive a vehicle that is easily accessible. If you do drive, you will need to take care that your hands, shoulders, neck, knees, and feet are mobile enough to operate a vehicle safely. If you have limited mobility, you may wish to have devices installed in the vehicle that make it easier to operate. Such devices are hand controls, foot controls, extra mirrors, wing mirrors, and panoramic mirrors.

Care should be taken that sidewalks, stairs, and driveways are free of ice and clutter so you will not slip or trip. Cars or trucks that are high off the ground can be a problem for people who have difficulty with their knees and hips. It may also be hard for you to use your hands to grip the edges of the doors and pull yourself up to get in. If the vehicle is high off the ground, use a stepstool to make entry easier.

For people with rheumatoid arthritis who live in cold climates, ice and snow can be very hazardous and treacherous to walk on, and the cold can cause the pain to increase, making movement difficult and painful. In warm climates, there is the advantage of no snow, ice, and cold but heat can cause the handles of doors and railings to become hot to the touch. If you have a problem with balance, grabbing a sun-scorched object for stability could cause injury. Placing padding or duct tape around metal handles and knobs will alleviate this problem.

Step height and ease of entry are considerations that people with disabilities have when using public transportation. If bus steps are too high or if the bus stop is too far away, then a cab or private service is required. Most communities have accessible transportation for people with physical limitations as part of the public transportation system. Some community and health centers provide transportation for a fee. One good resource to contact is the Easter Seals Foundation at www.easter-seals.org. Easter Seals has partnered with the American Bus Association to provide transportation for people with disabilities.

Parking is another issue. If the distance from the car to the health club, hospital pool, or public pool is too far, then you probably will not go. Before joining a club or community facility, investigate parking and ask if there is handicapped parking available and investigate getting a handicapped sticker for your car.

Building Access

Access to the building where there is a pool is important. Stairs and the distance from the parking lot to the door or the distance between the locker room and the pool within the building may be a problem. If you have trouble climbing stairs, you will need to find out how far the elevator is from the pool and the locker room. You will need to see if the locker room itself is large and roomy enough and if there are railings and supports along the walls. The locker room should be kept warm so muscles do not tighten up after getting out of the water. You should not use a facility that is hard to get to from the outside and hard to negotiate from the inside, no matter how wonderful the pool might be. If access is inconvenient, then the initiative to get out and exercise will disappear. Find a better location.

Clothing

Wearing the proper clothing in the pool is important for safety and comfort. Women and men should both wear swimsuits that fit properly. An ill-fitting suit, besides being uncomfortable, will fill with water and add additional weight. This causes drag, so when you shift direction, you could lose your balance. Drag from the water is desirable in an exercise program, but the person, not the swimsuit

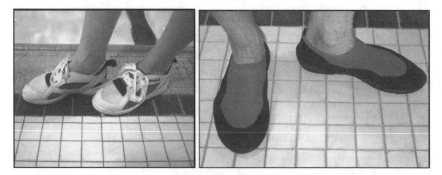

Figure 10: Water shoes that tie (left) and water shoes that slip on (right).

should have control over the drag force. Furthermore, if you wear a suit that is too tight or small, you might experience movement restriction and/or circulation problems. You need to be mindful of how a swimsuit will be put on and taken off and how this affects your ability to move, considering stiff fingers and possibly lack of hip and knee flexibility. Wear suits with simple closures that slip on and off easily rather than suits with complicated closures.

When exercising in a pool, it is advisable to wear water shoes. Many sporting goods stores sell these shoes. The shoes look like other exercise shoes, but they are made to withstand the water, and have perforations so water can easily drain out. Water shoes are water and chlorine resistant and are made of material such as neoprene. You will want shoes that have Velcro closures, drawstring closures, or that pull on easily. Shoes add stability and traction in the water and protect the tender soles of the feet in and out of the water. See Figure 10.

Goggles are optional. Some people are very sensitive to the chlorine levels used in pools. Their eyes may become irritated even if their head is not under the water. If you choose to wear goggles, you need to make sure you can see clearly out of them. Many goggles are made with lenses that are resistant to fogging. Polyvinyl or other soft foam material around the lenses allows the goggles to fit snugly against the skin, providing more comfort. Ordinary sunglasses sometimes work just as well.

If you exercise in an outdoor pool, a lightweight T-shirt may be worn for comfort and protection from the sun. It is important to wear

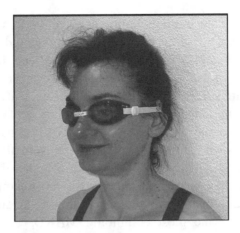

Figure 11: Goggles.

a well-fitting T-shirt that is not too loose or else the shirt can get tangled in some of the equipment or cause an unnatural drag effect. It is also advisable to use sunscreen and to wear a hat. Sunburn will do more than interfere with a good workout.

People with arthritis need to keep warm. If the pool water is too cool, a T-shirt may provide enough insulation to keep warm. Once you begin to move, your body will warm up. If you have Raynaud's phenomenon, latex surgical gloves, water gloves, and shoes will insulate your hands and feet from cold water.

Medications

A fitness trainer or physical therapist needs to know what kinds of medications you are taking before recommending a program. A description of the basic types of medications used for rheumatoid arthritis is provided. There is always new information coming out about new medications so it is important to stay current.

NSAIDs are used for people with rheumatoid arthritis to reduce inflammation and pain. The most common NSAIDs used by people with rheumatoid arthritis are aspirin and ibuprofen, COX-2 Inhibitors, NO-NSAIDs, DMARDs, and Corticosteroids. Although acetaminophen (Tylenol), or opioids such as Codeine, may reduce pain, they do not reduce inflammation as effectively as aspirin. If pain is reduced but not inflammation, more damage could be done to the joint. These medications have the same side effects for people with rheumatoid arthritis as they do for people with osteoarthritis.

DMARDs are specific to rheumatoid arthritis. DMARD stands for disease-modifying anti-rheumatic drugs. They are also known as slow-acting anti-rheumatic drugs or SAARDs. Both DMARDs and SAARDs slow down the progression of rheumatoid arthritis. Many of these drugs were originally used for conditions other than rheumatoid arthritis. When they were first studied for the treatment of cancer, researchers found that they were also helpful against rheumatoid arthritis. Some of the most common DMARDs are Methotrexate, Hydroxychloroquine, Sulfasalazine, gold, D-penicillamine, Cyclosporine, and Leflunomide. People with rheumatoid arthritis use DMARDs for only one or two years because they tend to lose their effectiveness. In order to extend the benefits of DMARDs, they are combined with other DMARDs or with different drugs such as corticosteroids. All DMARDs and SAARDs can cause stomach and intestinal side effects but in the long run these side effects may not be as severe as with NSAIDs.

Gold compounds contain gold in chemical form and can be administered as a pill or can be injected. Until the 1980s, gold treatment was the best relief available for people with rheumatoid arthritis. Gold treatment, sometimes referred to as gold salts, relieves joint pain and stiffness, reduces swelling, and reduces bone damage. Side effects include tongue irritation; skin rashes or itching; sore, red, or bleeding gums; diarrhea; and nausea. Some brand names for gold treatment include Ridaura, Solganal, and Myochrisine.

Rituximab, co-owned by Roche and Genentech Inc., is the newest drug to be tested. Trials of this new drug show that it is safe and effective plus cheaper and simpler to take than some of the other drugs. Rituximab is injected into the affected joints. Other drugs that are injected cause temporary reduction of symptoms but last only a week or two at the most, and the yearly cost of these injections is about $15,500. Rituximab costs around $6,200 for two injections and causes a temporary remission that can last for one to three years.

Professor Jo Edwards of University College London has been

conducting trials with Rituximab on patients with rheumatoid arthritis. Of 122 people injected twice with Rituximab, 80% had noticeable improvement of their rheumatoid arthritis condition. The side effects of Rituximab are similar to other drugs used to treat autoimmune diseases. These drugs attack the part of the immune system that is malfunctioning and this can leave the body in an immune deficient state and vulnerable to other illnesses. Edwards hopes the drug can be available in two to three years but until then, more trials and tests are needed to make sure Rituximab is truly safe.

It is not possible to list all of the medications that are available for people with arthritis. A good resource for fitness trainers, physical therapists, and people with arthritis is *Arthritis Medicines A-Z* by Dr. C. Michael Stein. Dr Stein's book is well organized and easy to understand. The medications are listed alphabetically by the generic name. Once the generic name is found, the brand names, type of arthritis it treats, dosage, side effects, and interactions with other medication are all listed.

4

Equipment

As you progress in your water exercise program, you should consider looking for some special equipment to use during the exercise program. All of the equipment discussed in this section can be purchased from fitness stores or can be ordered through the Internet. Many health clubs and rehabilitation centers have some or all of these items and will generally allow people to use them.

Some of the equipment, such as gloves, water weights, paddles, ankle weights, and noodles, are resistance equipment. They will make the exercises more strenuous as flexibility, endurance, and mobility are increased. Other equipment such as kickboards and jogging belts, make exercises easier by relieving pressure on the legs and back. Here are the most common types of water exercise equipment.

Water Gloves (Figure 12)

Water gloves are made of neoprene or chlorine resistant Lycra and have webbing between the fingers. This allows the hands to grab, push or pull more water and therefore gain more resistance and intensity. The gloves either slip on or have a Velcro clasp at the wrist. These are especially good for people who are suffering from flare-ups and have trouble holding onto free weights.

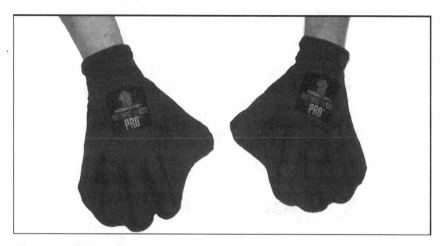

Figure 12: Water gloves

Water Weights (Figure 13)

Water weights look like dumbbells or barbells but are made of closed cell EVA foam. These are more durable than Styrofoam and the plates are non-abrasive. The bar between the plates is padded to help reduce over-gripping, which can be especially painful for people with arthritis. Dumbbells are held in each hand and barbells are held with both hands. Barbells are 25" to 30" in length. Some barbells have a curved bar to allow for better hand positioning. Dumbbells and barbells come in varying weights and sizes. They are feather light on land but are resistant to pushing down in the water since they are

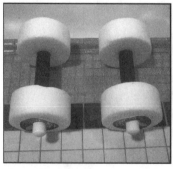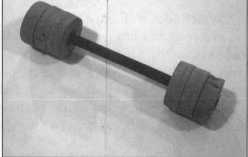

Figure 13: Water weights, dumbbells, and barbell

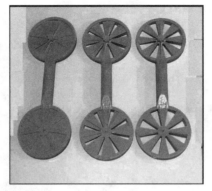

Figure 14: Paddles

buoyant. By manipulating the dumbbells under water, you gain the same level of resistance training that a weight trainer has when using metal dumbbells on land. The dumbbells and barbells are used mostly to help strengthen the upper body, arms, chest, torso, and back.

Paddles (Figure 14)

Paddles are plastic dumbbells that have pinwheels at the ends instead of Styrofoam plates. The paddles provide resistance when dragged through the water. The pinwheels are adjustable and can be opened for less resistance, allowing water to flow through the wheel, or closed, allowing for more resistance. It is advisable to start with paddles before progressing to water weights or noodles.

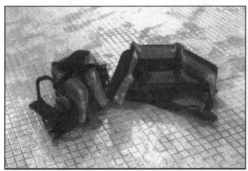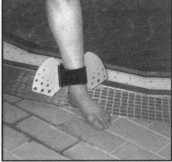

Figure 15: Ankle weights and water wings

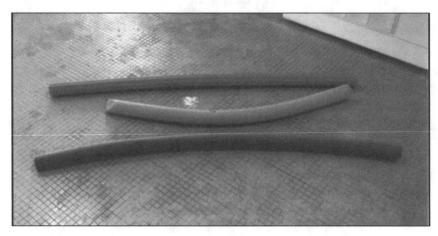

Figure 16: Noodles

Ankle Weights and Water Wings (Figure 15)

Ankle weights and water wings are cuffs made for both the wrist and the ankle. They are made of soft santoprene rubber or nylon covered Styrofoam. They provide both drag and buoyant resistance like water weights. Since they are strapped onto the body, they are easier to control than water weights. For the beginner who may not be used to any type of water equipment, it might be easier to start with ankle weights, water wings, or paddles. Once these pieces of equipment have been mastered, then you can try water weights.

Noodles (Figure 16)

Noodles are long cylindrical tubes made of Styrofoam. They were originally made as flotation toys for children. There are two types of noodles, one is hollow and the other is a solid tube. The hollow tube is easier to manipulate. Both types come in varying lengths. Again, by manipulating the tube underwater, you are able to increase the water resistance. The noodles are used for strengthening the legs, abdominal work, and to stabilize and enhance your balance.

Kickboards (Figure 17)

Kickboards are buoyant, durable, lightweight, flat boards that you can use to support yourself while performing exercises in the water. The most common type of exercise that uses a kickboard is one where

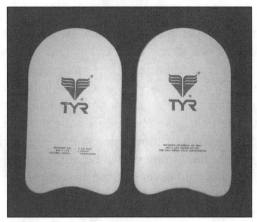

Figure 17: Kickboards

you are prone in the water.

Jogging Belt (Figure 18)
The jogging belt is used to raise your body off the floor of the

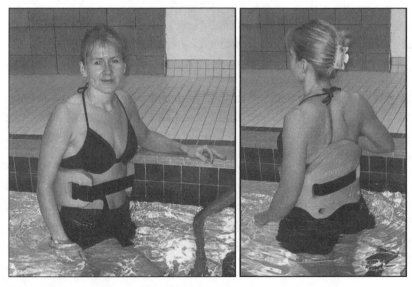

Figure 18: Jogging belt, front and back

pool and keep you in a vertical position. The belts come in different styles. Some are wide, sculpted EVA foam belts and others are made of foam blocks that are strung on a nylon belt. The wide, sculpted belts are more expensive and offer a little more security.

The jogging belt can be used in water as shallow as chest deep. This is a helpful piece of equipment for a person with sore knees, ankles, or feet. The belt lifts your body's weight off the joints while still allowing for freedom of movement to run, jog, or bicycle in the water. It is very important to understand that the jogging belt is not a flotation device and should never be used as such.

Equipment for People with Advanced Arthritis

For people who have advanced osteoarthritis or rheumatoid arthritis there is equipment such as full body floating mats, splints, canes, and aquatic wheel chairs.

Full body floating mats are good for people who have limited mobility in large areas of their body. The mat can be used to support the area that has limited movement while you exercise the more available body areas. For example, if you are disabled in the hips and knees, you can lie prone on the mat and exercise your arms, shoulders, and back.

Splints can be worn to protect very sensitive joints. While the ever-present movement of the water is great for regaining balance, it can be a problem if a joint is so sore it shouldn't be moved. Splints can help with this concern.

A cane made of water resistant material can give you a better sense of balance and security, if you need it. When using a cane, you should be careful not to use one that is too high. A cane that is too high may upset your balance.

Aquatic Wheelchairs (Figure 19)

Most pool facilities that specialize in programs for people with physical limitations provide aquatic wheelchairs. A person with limited mobility is still able to do upper body and lower body strengthening exercises from an aquatic wheelchair.

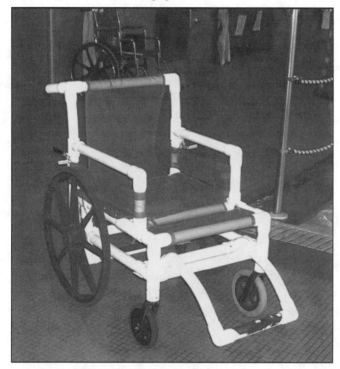

Figure 19: Aquatic wheel chair

It is a good idea to look for a facility that supplies this equipment as part of its program. It will save you some money and it is a good indication that the facility is committed to providing good programs for people with physical limitations.

5

The Exercise Companion

This chapter is for people who are helping someone with arthritis participate in a water exercise program. It is important that the participant and the companion each understand their roles and their relationship. When people work out together, they do so in order to help motivate and support one another in their desire to get fit. When one of the participants has arthritis, he or she may require more monitoring and attention than the more able-bodied companion. Even though the able-bodied companion will want to have an effective workout, the primary responsibility of the companion is to offer support to the person with arthritis. It is important that the companion be aware of what arthritis is and know a little about how to assess the partner's condition and abilities. The companion can assist the person with arthritis with passive and active assistive stretches and can provide moral support and encouragement.

When working with a person who has arthritis, it is important to be sensitive when referring to the participant. Avoid references to the person with arthritis as "victim," "sufferer," or "handicapped." Instead, use the term "disability," or perhaps don't mention it at all. Do not portray people with arthritis who are successful as superhuman. This implies that other people who have disabilities are unsuccessful. Avoid using negative phrases such as "confined to a wheelchair." Instead use positive references such as "uses a wheelchair."

People with arthritis can have a number of psychosocial issues. They include: loneliness, fear of being deformed and/or disabled, an uncertain future, helplessness and dependency, financial difficulties, worries about physical barriers caused by their disability, worries about other peoples' attitudes towards them, and anger and grief over the change in their body and how it impacts their life and lifestyle. If the person with arthritis is hearing impaired or visually impaired, there may be additional anger, depression, and resentment. This will be an additional challenge for the companion.

The companion can offer an increased feeling of well-being, which helps to decrease the onset of depression, gives the person with arthritis a sense of purpose, and alleviates feelings of isolation. The companion can encourage and motivate the person to exercise and make it a lifelong habit.

Whether the companion is a personal friend, family member, physical therapist, or water fitness instructor, the method of communication is important. Communication is the act of sending information. Verbal communication uses words and sounds to create meaning. Nonverbal communication uses bodily gestures or props to convey a message. Part of nonverbal communication uses emblems and illustrators as methods of conveying a message. Emblems are defined as bodily cues that are easy to translate verbally and their meaning is precise. Illustrators are defined as use of the arms, hands, and head to help increase the clarity of verbal messages. The use of emblems and illustrators when teaching water fitness to a group or an individual becomes a dialog of sign language between the instructor and the participant(s). The participant(s) must be able to understand the message sent by the companion as well as the companion being able to understand the participant is receiving the message. The face is used more than any other part of the body to convey the intensity of the messages being sent, whether verbally or nonverbally.

Both verbal and nonverbal communications are important when working in the water with a person who has arthritis. It is not only important to verbally describe an exercise; it is also important to visually demonstrate the exercise so the person with arthritis can perform the movement correctly keeping the person with arthritis informed about the benefits of a particular exercise.

When helping with an exercise program, the companion and the person with arthritis must address:

- General flexibility or range of motion.
- Stretching with relaxation
- Balance and posture
- Endurance
- Strength

An exercise program should consist of flexibility training, endurance training, and strength training. The companion needs to assess if the person with arthritis can stretch effectively and determine if the person is flexible and strong enough to engage in strength training and endurance training. The exercise program should have elements that address each of these areas and the companion's role is to ensure that these areas are actually performed by the person with arthritis.

Relaxation is important as a way to reduce problems with muscle stiffness. Exercises that help induce relaxation include stretching and deep breathing.

Balance and posture are important because maintaining an upright posture helps the person with arthritis to move and walk more efficiently with less stress on the joints. When people with arthritis experience muscle atrophy due to a lack of exercise, the decreased muscle strength allows gravity to pull the body forward. This increases postural instability that can lead to falls. Having the body lean forward over the knees puts excess pressure on the joints causing further cartilage damage. Stooped posture also inhibits the diaphragm, which needs to expand for proper breathing. Some of the exercises that can help with postural maintenance include March with a Kick, Side to Side Step, and Arm Cross.

Flexibility training concentrates on increasing range of motion (ROM). Range of motion is important because it improves ease and fluidity of movement. Working on flexibility reduces stiffness and muscle atrophy. Some of the exercises that help with ROM are hip exercises, shoulder flexibility/ROM exercises, trunk and neck exercises. These can be found in Chapters 8 and 9.

Endurance training is achieved with exercises that lead to a better functioning heart, lungs, and circulatory system. Exercises that help with endurance are The Water Jog, Knee Lift with a Kick, and any of the aerobic exercises found in Chapter 10.

Strength training is important so the muscles retain their ability to move the body. Strong muscles improve joint stability and makes movements easier and safer to perform. The strength exercises are found in Chapter 11.

6

Preparing to Exercise

A well-rounded exercise program consists of six main components: warm-ups, flexibility training (also known as range of motion or ROM), stretching, aerobic training (also known as cardiovascular or endurance training), strength training, and cool down. The types of arthritis you have and the amount of pain and inflammation you are experiencing on a particular day will determine how much of each component you will be able to perform.

The breakdown of a typical exercise session depends on the type of arthritis. For people who have rheumatoid arthritis an equal amount of aerobics and strength training along with warm-ups and stretching is appropriate. The cardiovascular conditioning helps keep the ratio of fat and muscle in the proper proportion and the strengthening exercises help keep the muscles in good condition. The schedule would typically have:

- 5-10 minutes of warm-up exercises
- 5-10 minutes of flexibility exercises
- 5-10 minutes of stretching exercises
- 15-25 minutes of aerobic activity at an appropriate intensity level
- 5 minutes of lower intensity level aerobics
- 15-25 minutes of strength training exercises
- 5 minutes of a cool down which is like the warm-up exercises, but less intense
- 5 minutes of stretching

At the beginning of an exercise session, the warm-up exercises prepare the joints and muscles by getting them moving and warmed-up, allowing the synovial fluid to lubricate the joints. The flexibility and range of motion exercises get the stabilizer muscles warmed up. Going through the flexibility exercises at an increasing pace allows you to move right into the stretches. The stretching exercises elongate the mobilizer muscles to give more range of motion.

The aerobic part of the exercise session consists of movements that are continuous, fluid, and intense for an extended time. After an appropriate amount of time, the pace slows down for a few minutes to allow the heart rate to come down gradually.

The strengthening part of the program is next. If you have swelling in the joints from rheumatoid arthritis, you may want to omit or modify this part of the program.

Strength training can be incorporated into the aerobic session through the use of water gloves and ankle weights. As you engage in the aerobic session, the addition of water equipment provides added resistance so the arms and legs are also being strengthened.

You should try to perform each exercise correctly to its full potential. A partner or fitness trainer can monitor your progress through effective, positive, visual and verbal cueing. Before increasing the intensity or repetitions of any of the exercises, you should be able to comfortably perform the exercises at a constant level for four to five days. Once that level of proficiency has been obtained, you may want to be challenged by more repetitions and/or more intensity.

It is important to stretch before and after each exercise session. Stretching is an essential element in maintaining and improving flexibility. Deep breathing exercises will also help you relax after exercising.

After exercising, you need to relax. This is time set aside for personal, physical, and emotional improvement. You need to feel as healthy as possible both inside and outside. It is important for you to remember you are in control of your destiny so you are not a burden to yourself or other family members and friends. One of the most important aspects of preparing to exercise is to understand that it is worth the time and the effort.

7

Warm-Ups

Before doing any exercises, you should take at least five minutes to warm up your muscles. There are several warm-ups described in this chapter. Warm-ups start with loosening up the lower body and then move to the upper body. The warm-ups include slow, stationary movements for the legs and arms along with a mix of gentle stretching. Warming up the muscles increases blood flow and helps to prevent injuries.

There are numerous full body warm-ups that are good for you. When performing these warm-ups you should check and recheck your posture. Correct posture involves positioning the pelvis so the back has a normal curve. The pelvis should not tip too far forward pushing the gluteus up and out nor should the pelvis tip back causing the gluteus to tuck to far under the body. This is called neutral posture. Good posture whether standing, sitting, lying, or walking, allow you to function effectively without straining the muscles, tendon, ligaments, and joints.

When standing, keep your chin parallel to the pool floor; keep your feet shoulder-width apart and your toes pointed slightly outward. Press your shoulders back and down and let your arms hang loosely down by the sides of your body. Try to make all of the arm and leg motions as smoothly and rhythmically as possible and breathe easily throughout the exercise. These warm-ups work the muscles of the arms, chest, back, hips, and knees.

Water Cycle is especially good for people who have rheumatoid arthritis because the body is suspended by the jogging belt and the water surrounds and cushions the lower body so any inflamed joints do not experience painful pressure while the muscles are being put through a full range of motion.

During the performance of any of the warm-ups, you may stand near enough to the pool edge to be able to grab the pool wall for support.

Walking with Swinging Arms

This warm-up works best when it is done in water that is chest deep. Walk about 50 feet while swinging both arms from the shoulder. The palms should be turned up to lift the water, thus using the resistance of the water to make the exercise a little more challenging. If this position puts too much pressure on the shoulder joint, keep your arms closer to the side of the body. While walking in this manner, you need to concentrate on lifting your legs from the hip joint, rolling your body weight from the heel to the toe of each foot, distributing your weight evenly between your feet so you avoid shuffling.

The arms can swing in two different ways. The first is an alternating fashion with one arm swinging to the front and one arm swinging to the back. Note that the arm swinging forward and the front leg are on the same side, not the way we usually walk. The second arm movement is to swing both arms up and back at the same time. This will change your center of gravity so you will need to keep your posture steady and upright and the core muscles flexed. This walk warms the muscles of the arms, chest, back, hips, legs, and feet.

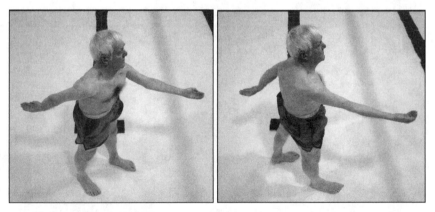

Figure 20: Walking with Swinging Arms, alternating arms

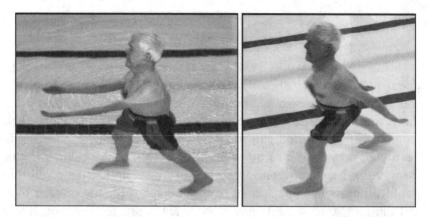

Figure 21: Walking with Swinging Arms, matching arms

The March

The March is a stationary warm-up. While standing in waist to chest deep water, lift your knee to hip level then lower your leg and repeat the movement with the other leg. The muscles being warmed up are the hips, buttocks, thighs, and calves. You may want to stand close to the pool edge so you can use the edge for balance.

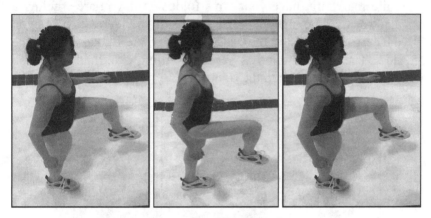

Figure 22: The March

March with Rocking Arms

Standing in water that is waist to chest deep, create a marching motion by lifting one knee so the thigh is parallel to the pool floor and then return the leg to a standing position. Then the other knee is lifted and lowered. The march is done in an alternating fashion for about 50 feet. This warm-up may also be done in place.

While marching, have your arms folded as if you are cradling a baby and rocking the imaginary baby in a side-to-side motion. As you lift your left knee, twist at the waist and move the folded arms to the left side. Then this motion is repeated lifting the right knee and swinging the folded arms to the right side.

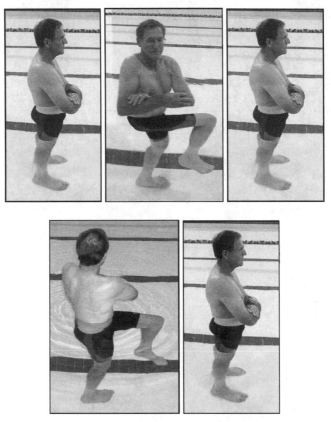

Figure 23: March with Rocking Arms, rocking to the same side

If it is difficult for you to twist your upper body to the same side as the lifted knee, you may bring the arms to the opposite side. You should start with small steps and gradually work up to a moderate pace to warm up the legs, hips, back, shoulders, and torso.

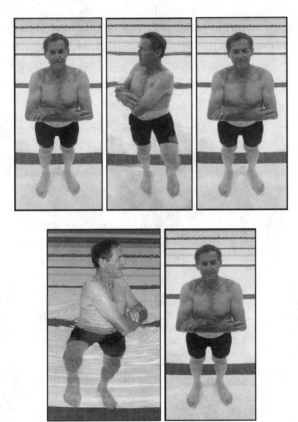

Figure 24: March with Rocking Arms, front view, rocking to the opposite side

March with a Kick

While standing in waist to chest deep water, march in place or move through the water. Your knee is brought up to hip level so that the thigh is parallel to the pool floor. The lower leg is then extended outward. After returning the straightened leg to the pool bottom, repeat the exercise with the other leg. If lowering the leg with a straight knee puts too much strain on your back or hips, the knee can be bent again before the leg is lowered. This warm-up affects the hips, buttocks, thighs, and calves.

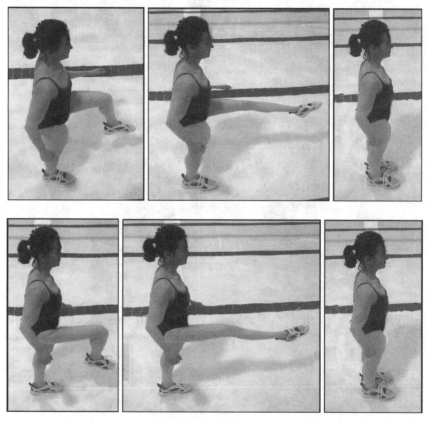

Figure 25: March with a Kick

Ice Skating

This warm-up can be performed in waist to chest deep water. Step out in a forward motion and slowly transfer your weight from the back foot to the front foot taking four to eight counts for the transfer. Then the other foot is placed in front and the weight is transferred slowly to the front leg. Continue alternating from one leg to the other. While skating, reach forward with the arm on the same side as the leg that is supporting the body's weight. The muscles being warmed-up are the shoulders, back, hips, knees, and feet. Avoid placing too much pressure on the knee joint, especially of the knee is inflamed or painful.

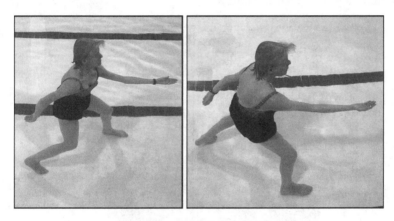

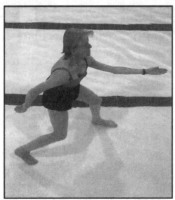

Figure 26: Ice Skating

Walking with American Crawl Arms

Stand in chest deep water close enough to the pool wall for comfort and support. As you walk in a circle or the width of the pool, rotate the arms from the shoulders as if you are doing the American crawl swimming stroke. To start, the arms are extended out front with the palms facing down. As you walk, the right arm swings down from the shoulder and reaches as far back as is comfortable. Turn the palm up and bring the arm up out of the water and then, with the palm rotated down, the arm is returned to the water. As the right arm gets about halfway through its rotation, the left arm begins its cycle. This alternating circle pattern with the arms continues as you walk continuously in the same manner.

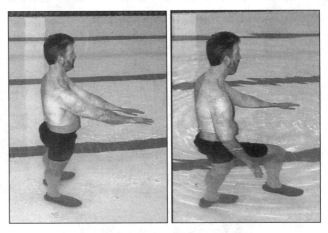

Figure 27: Walking with American Crawl Arms

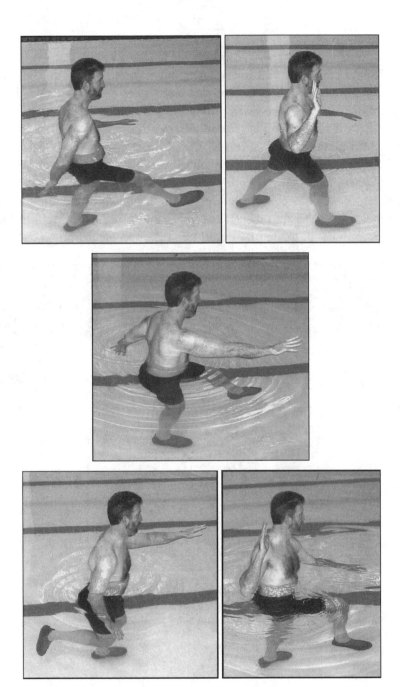

Figure 28: Walking with American Crawl Arms, continued

Side to Side Step

This exercise is good for balance and warms up the hip joints in the sagittal plane. Stand in waist to chest deep water with the legs together. You should be facing the pool wall and be close enough to reach it for balance, if it is required. Bring the left leg up, bent at the knee, and place the left foot down off to the side of the body. This will require you to balance momentarily on your right foot until the left foot is placed on the pool floor. Once the left foot is down, the right leg moves close to the left leg again. The step to the left should be repeated four to six times. Then you should step to the right in the same way for four to six times until you return to the starting location.

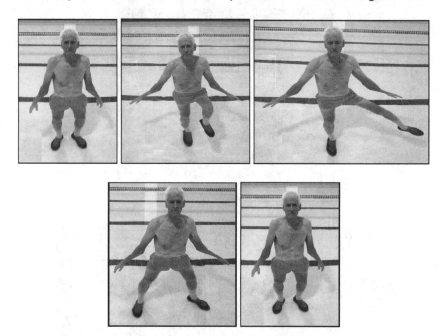

Figure 29: Side to Side Step, moving left

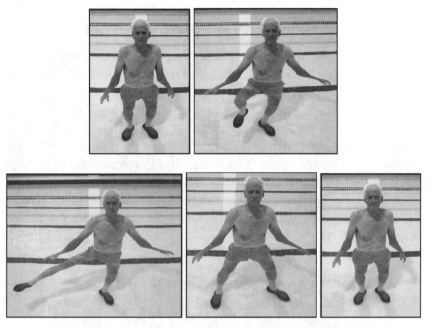

Figure 30: Side to Side Step, moving right

Walking with Breaststroke Arms

Stand in chest deep water. The starting position is with the elbows out to the side, hands close to the chest, and palms of the hands parallel to each other and close together. To do the exercise, walk a short distance back and forth or in a small circle. As you walk, you push your hands forward. Rotate the hands at the wrist so the palms face outward, then attempt to part the water in a breaststroke. The stroke is completed when your arms circle around and are brought back to the starting position. This water walk can be done with the assistance of a companion or you can stay close to the pool edge for balance. This walk warms the muscles of the arms, chest, back, hips, legs, and feet.

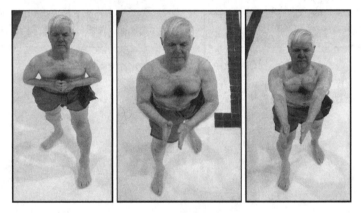

Figure 31: Walking with Breaststroke Arms, beginning

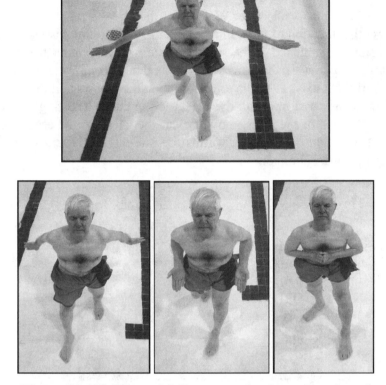

Figure 32: Walking with Breaststroke Arms, continued

Walking with Rowing Arms

Perform this walk like Walking with Breaststroke Arms but reverse the direction of the arm movement. While doing this walk, the arms start outstretched at the sides and are held just under the water surface. As you walk the arms swing around and scoop water with the palms of the hands. Then the arms fold in at the elbows and the hands fold in at the wrist bringing the hands to the chest. The fingers then follow the line of the arms, moving near the chest, as the arms open up to begin again. This walk warms the muscles of the arms, chest, back, hips, legs, and feet.

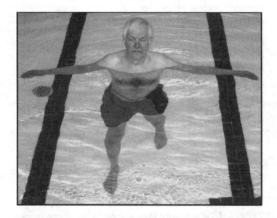

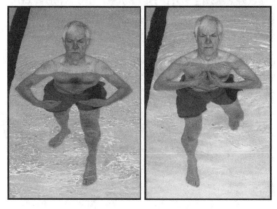

Figure 33: Walking with Rowing Arms

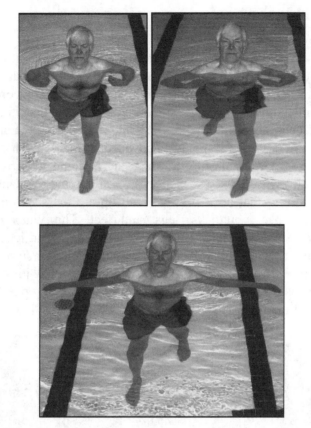

Figure 34: Walking with Rowing Arms, continued

The Water Cycle

This warm-up is best done while using a jogging belt. (Put it on before entering the pool.) Move to water that is deep enough so your feet don't touch the bottom of the pool. Once you are at a comfortable depth, gently move your legs in a circular motion that imitates the motion of peddling a bicycle. At the same time, swing the arms back and forth as if running slowly. The hands should be in a cupped position so they are able to grab the water, adding more resistance. You may also wish to use water gloves for additional resistance.

The muscles that are being warmed up are the shoulders, arms, wrist, chest, back, buttocks, legs, and feet. The Water Cycle is especially good if you have sore places in the hips and legs because the body is suspended by the jogging belt and the water surrounds and cushions the lower body. Tender points or inflamed joints do not experience painful pressure while the muscles are being put through a full range of motion.

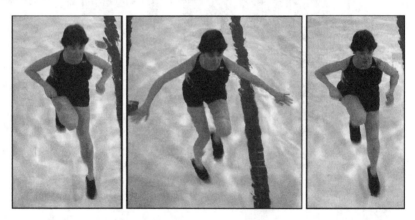

Figure 35: The Water Cycle using a jogging belt

The Water Cycle can also be done while being supported by a noodle. Wrap the noodle around your body and lie in a prone position on the noodle. A companion may stand behind you and help stabilize the noodle from behind making it easier for you to hold your head up, especially if you have stiffness or pain in your neck.

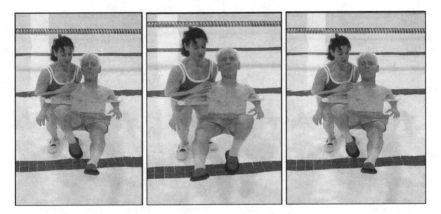

Figure 36: The Water Cycle using a noodle, with help from a companion

8

Flexibility and Range of Motion

One of the biggest problems you will have when you are dealing with rheumatoid arthritis is a tendency to tighten the muscles around a painful joint to keep it from moving. In the case of an acute injury, such as an ankle sprain, this is a useful response because it prevents additional injury. In the case of rheumatoid arthritis, the joint needs to move as freely as possible. Tightening up and limiting the movement only makes the condition worse.

In this chapter we will look at exercises that improve range of motion and flexibility by increasing your ability to move your joints freely. There are actually two aspects to being able to move easily, which are reflected in the two ways muscles are involved in movement. Some muscles, called mobilizers, cause the movement and others, called stabilizers, react to postural signals to keep the body in the proper position while moving.

Mobilizers are made of fast twitch fibers and are found close to the body's surface. They are long muscles that usually stretch the whole length of the bone, sometimes across two or more joints. An example would be the biceps, the muscle in the front of the upper arm. It attaches to the shoulder blade at the top and the forearm at the bottom and is responsible for flexing the elbow. Mobilizers are responsible for the body's ability to produce rapid movements or movements that require a lot of force.

Stabilizers are shorter muscles with less range of motion that are usually deeper under the body's surface. They attach across a single joint and are responsible for holding it in the proper alignment for movement, posture, and balance. Stabilizers are made up of slow-twitch fibers, so they don't react as quickly or with as much force, but they have much greater endurance. For example, stabilizer muscles in the shoulder keep the shoulder from moving when the biceps is flexing the elbow.

Both sets of muscles can become tight and restrict your movement, which also leads to greater pain. One pattern that is often seen is a joint with some muscles that are too tight and others that are too loose. The exercises in this chapter are designed to balance the muscles appropriately. Muscles that are too tight will be stretched through the movements and will increase their range of motion. Muscles that are too loose will be exercised by the resistance of the water and get stronger so they can do their job more effectively.

This chapter focuses mainly on stabilizer muscles. The next chapter on Stretching shows how to lengthen mobilizers.

Another aspect of flexibility is the joint capsule itself. Problems within the joint capsule, such as a lack of synovial fluid, can restrict flexibility as much as tight muscles. Happily these exercises are just the kind of gentle movement that stimulates production of synovial fluid and frees up the tissues in the joint capsule to allow you to move more easily.

It is important for you to consult with your physician before performing these flexibility exercises, especially if you have had surgery or if your joints are severely swollen.

You need to perform these motions in a slow and controlled manner, breathing easily and naturally, and performing the exercises through your full range, but not to the point of pain. If pain is experienced, you should stop and, if the pain persists, consult your physician. If possible, the exercises should be done daily. While doing the flexibility exercises, you may stand near to the edge of the pool so you can grab the pool wall for support, if you need to.

Pelvic Tilt

This flexibility exercise is for the lower back and helps to loosen and lengthen the spine. Stand in chest deep water leaning against the pool wall. Starting in a neutral position, rotate the pelvis forward so the hipbones start to face upward. Then gently tilt the pelvis back to a neutral position. It may help if you place one hand on the abdomen and one hand on the lower back so you are able to feel the movement. The pelvic tilt should be repeated four to eight times.

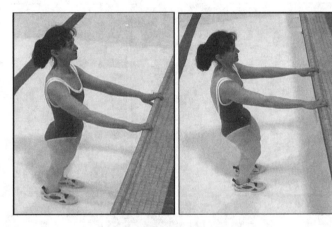

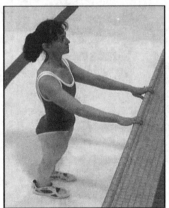

Figure 37: Pelvic Tilt

Hip Circles

This flexibility exercise loosens up the hips and lower back and helps with balance and posture. Stand in waist to chest deep water with your hands on your hips, feet shoulder width apart, and legs straight without locking the knees. Without moving the feet, rotate your pelvis in a clockwise circle four to six times and then reverse the circle and rotate your pelvis in a counterclockwise circle for four to six times.

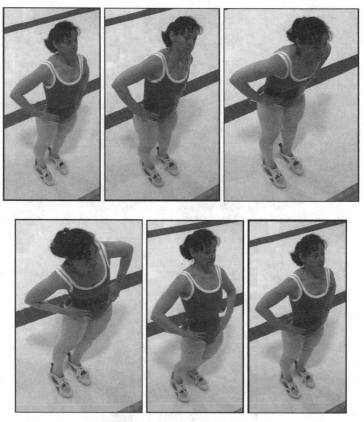

Figure 38: Hip Circles

Hips One

Stand in chest deep water with your back against the pool wall. Slowly tilt the pelvis forward and lift one knee to the chest and then return the knee to the starting position. Then lift the other knee toward the chest and return the knee to the starting position. These movements should be done in an alternating fashion slowly and smoothly for six to eight times on each side. This flexibility exercise warm-up is not recommended if you have had recent knee or hip surgery.

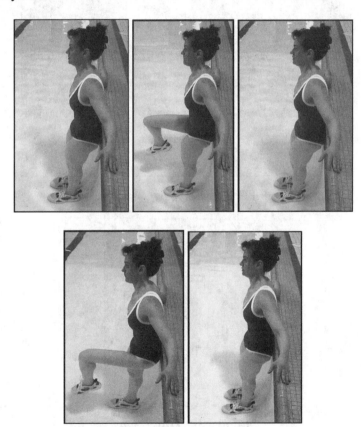

Figure 39: Hips One

Hips Two

Stand in chest deep water with your arm resting on the pool wall. Slowly lift one leg out to the side as much as possible, away from the midline of the body. Then bring the leg slowly back to the starting position. This motion should be repeated six to eight times with both the right and left legs.

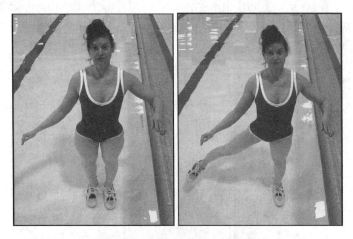

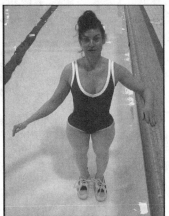

Figure 40: Hips Two

Hips Three

This flexibility exercise loosens the hip joint by rotating the femur bone inside the socket joint. Stand with your arm resting on the pool ledge in waist to chest deep water. Lift the heel of the leg farthest from the pool side towards the buttocks. The exercise is done by drawing a circle with the knee of the bent leg, keeping the knee pointed down. Start the circle toward the front and then move the knee away from the midline and around the circle until the knee is in back of the body. Then return it to the starting position. The complete circle should be done six to eight times. Make another six to eight circles with the knee starting toward the back (reversing the direction of the circle). After resting for a few seconds, the motion is repeated with the other leg.

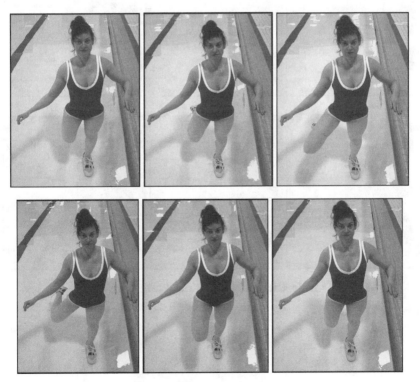

Figure 41: Hips Three

Ankle Circles

This is another flexibility exercise that can be done while sitting on the edge of the pool. Dangle your feet in the water, take one foot and extend it up at an angle, rotate the foot clockwise at the ankle eight to ten times and then rotate the foot counterclockwise eight to ten times. The ankle should move smoothly and evenly throughout the motion.

You can also perform the ankle circles by moving both ankles at the same time.

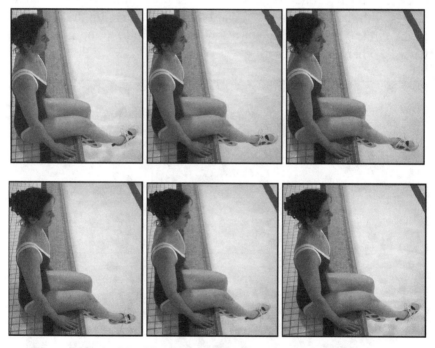

Figure 42: Ankle Circles, on the poolside with single ankles

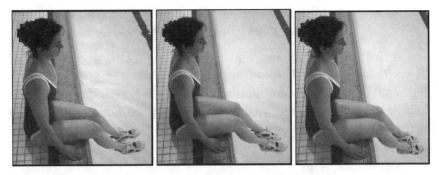

Figure 43: Ankle Circles, on the poolside with double ankles

An alternative way to perform this flexibility exercise is to stand in waist to chest deep water with one arm holding the pool ledge. One leg is lifted, suspending the foot in the water so it can be rotated at the ankle eight to ten times in a clockwise direction. Then reverse the motion and rotate the ankle counterclockwise eight to ten times. Then repeat this exercise with the other foot, making sure the support leg has a slightly bent knee.

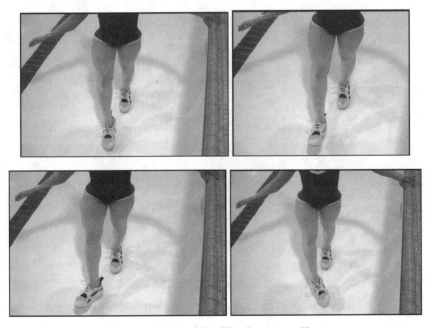

Figure 44: Ankle Circles, standing

Ankle Flexion and Extension

This flexibility exercise can be done sitting on the side of the pool or while standing in the pool. Sit on the edge of the pool with your legs dangling in the water and bend the lower leg 90 degrees. Point and flex the feet together or in an alternating fashion. This exercise helps to lubricate and loosen the ankle joint. Perform this movement eight to ten times.

An alternative way to perform this exercise is for you to stand in waist to chest deep water with your side to the pool wall, resting one arm on the ledge for support. Extend one leg out in front at the hip and flex and extend the foot at the ankle eight to ten times and then switch to the other foot. The foot may be suspended slightly off the pool floor. If balance is an issue, you may rest the heel of the foot gently on the pool floor. The leg that is supporting the weight should have a slight bend at the knee joint.

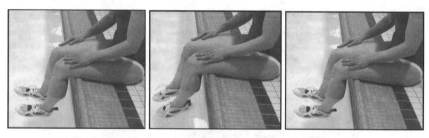

Figure 45: Ankle Flexion and Extension, on the pool side

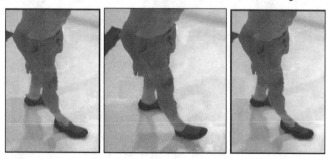

Figure 46: Ankle Flexion and Extension, standing

Knees

This flexibility exercise loosens the knee joint. Stand arm's length from pool wall in waist to chest deep water. Using the pool wall for support, stand with your legs close together. Bend slightly at the knee, then lift one leg up in back toward the buttocks making sure to keep your upper thighs still and perpendicular to the pool floor. Then place the leg back in the standing position and lift the other leg. This movement should be repeated in an alternating fashion for six to ten times. An alternative exercise would be to do six to eight repetitions with the right knee and then switch and do six to eight repetitions with the left knee.

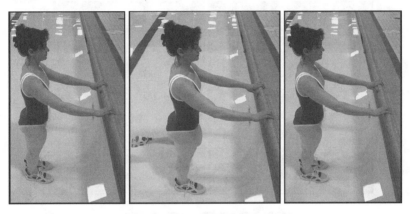

Figure 47: Knees

Toes

Standing in waist to chest deep water with arms on the side of the pool wall for stability, shift your weight to the left leg. With your right foot flat on the pool floor, curl the toes of the right foot and extend them. It is important that the toes are relaxed to prevent cramping in the foot. After repeating this movement six to ten times, shift your weight to the right leg and repeat the toe curl/extension with the toes of the left foot for six to ten counts. This flexibility exercise can also be done with both feet working at the same time. You can also sit on the stairs of the pool and perform this exercise.

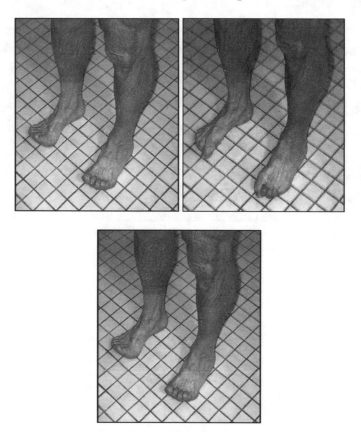

Figure 48: Toes

Shoulder Flexibility One

Shoulder rolls are good for preventing a rounded back and maintaining good posture. Shoulder rolls loosen and lubricate the shoulder joint, help to release tension within the neck and shoulders, and help to maintain a full range of motion. Stand in chest deep water and lift the shoulders upwards, forward, and down four to six times. The movement is then reversed by rolling the shoulders back away from the ears and lowering them down as if to set them into pockets in the back. This exercise is repeated four to six times and movements should be made in smooth, continuous circular motions.

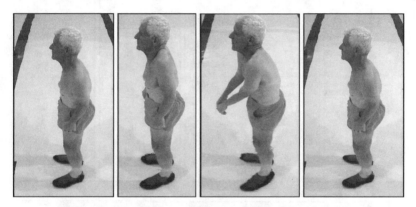

Figure 49: Shoulder Flexibility One, rolling forward

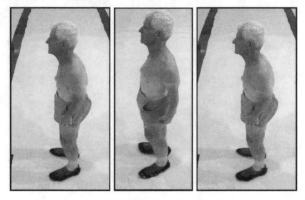

Figure 50: Shoulder Flexibility One, rolling backward

Shoulder Flexibility Two

This flexibility exercise concentrates on the anterior and posterior muscles of the shoulder. Stand in chest deep water, arm's length from the pool wall, with your arms alongside your body. Slowly raise your arms up in front as high as you can, keeping the palms up and in a cupped position. Then turn the palms down and lower the arms pulling them back behind your body as far as possible.

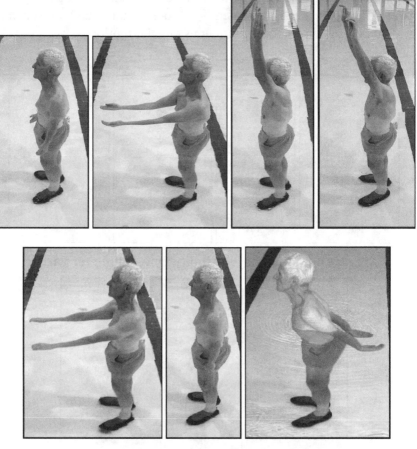

Figure 51: Shoulder Flexibility Two

Shoulder Flexibility Three

This flexibility exercise concentrates on the medial muscle of the shoulder. Stand in chest deep water, arm's length from the pool wall, with your arms alongside your body. Starting with the arms at the sides of the body, lift the arms out to the side and then up as far as you can with the palms up. Then turning the palms down, return the arms to the sides of the body and repeat this motion six to eight times.

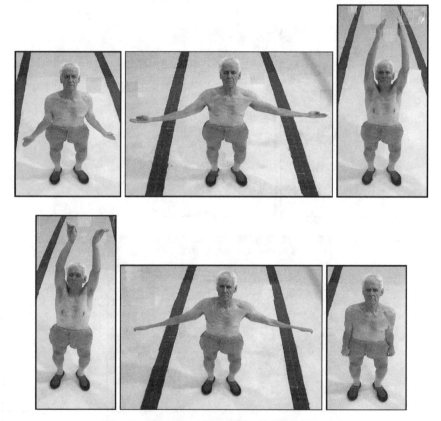

Figure 52: Shoulder Flexibility Three

Middle and Upper Back One

This flexibility exercise helps to improve range of motion and posture. Stand straight up in waist to chest deep water. The arms are relaxed and along the sides of the body. Bend at the waist and slowly slide your right hand down the right leg as far as it is comfortable. Once you have reached the maximum point of stretch, slowly reverse the movement until you have returned to an upright posture. This is then repeated with the left side. Do two to six repetitions on each side.

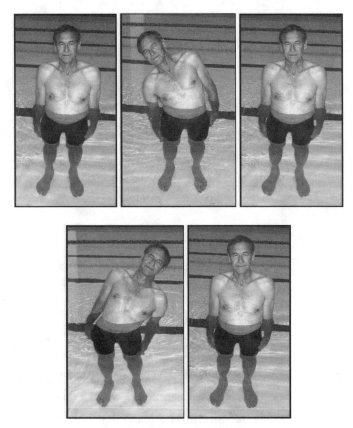

Figure 53: Middle and Upper Back One

Middle and Upper Back Two

This flexibility exercise helps to improve range of motion and posture. Stand in water that is waist to chest deep with your feet shoulder width apart and arms crossed at the chest. While tilting the pelvis forward, tightening the abdomen, and keeping the hips still, slowly turn your head and torso to the left side as far as is comfortable and then slowly turn to the right side. It is important that the head and upper body stay aligned. This rotation should be repeated four to six times.

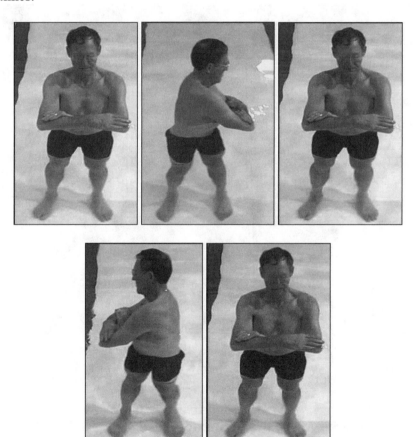

Figure 54: Middle and Upper Back Two

Arms, Breast Stroke

Sitting or standing in chest deep water push your hands forward. Then rotate your hands at the wrist so your palms face outward and part the water as in a breaststroke. The stroke is completed when the arms circle around and are brought to the starting position. The movement should be repeated six to ten times. This flexibility exercise can be done while standing or while sitting on the pool steps, on a water board, or a noodle.

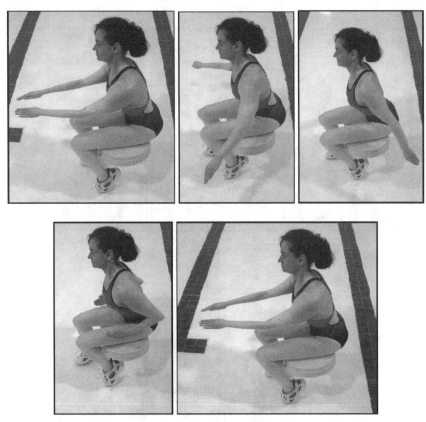

Figure 55: Arms, Breast Stroke, seated on a kick board

Arms, Rowing

Sit or stand in chest deep water with arms outstretched at the sides, just under the water surface. Bring the arms around in front, scooping the water with the palms of the hands and then fold the arms in at the elbows and the hands in at the wrist. Then pull the arms towards the chest. The fingers follow the line of the arms as the arms open up to go back to the original position. This flexibility exercise can be done while you are standing or while you sit on the pool stairs, a noodle, or a water board. This rowing motion should be repeated for six to ten repetitions.

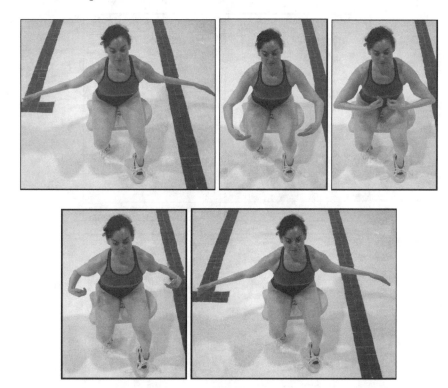

Figure 56: Arms, Rowing, seated on a kick board

Arms, American Crawl

With the arms extended out front and the palms facing down, stand or sit in chest deep water. Swing the right arm down from the shoulder and pull the arm back as far back as is comfortable. The palm is then turned up and the arm is brought out of the water. Then with the palm again rotated down, the arm is returned to the water. Repeat this alternating circle pattern with the left arm in a continuous pattern for six to ten repetitions. This flexibility exercise can be done while you are standing or sitting on the pool stairs, a noodle, or a water board.

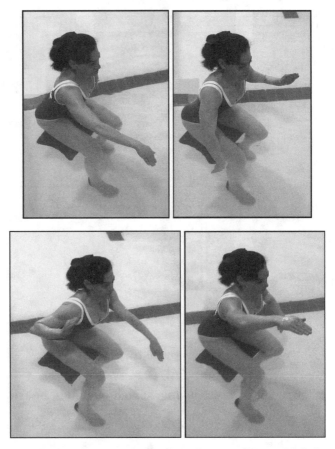

Figure 57: Arms, American Crawl, seated on a kick board

Elbows

This flexibility exercise prepares the elbow joint for biceps and triceps moves. Stand in chest deep water in a neutral position with your arms at your sides and palms facing up. Bring the fingers of both hands up to the shoulders with the palms facing the body. Then turning the palms to face outward, move the arms back to a straight position. The elbows stay at the sides the whole time. This exercise should be repeated six to ten times.

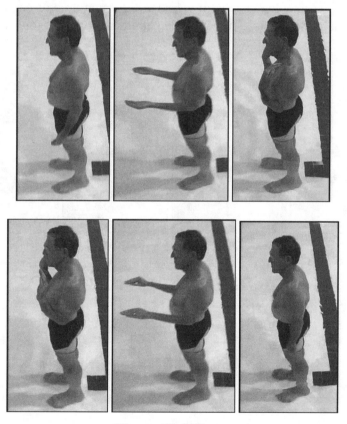

Figure 58: Elbows

Wrist Flexion and Extension

This flexibility exercise loosens up the wrist joint and warms up the muscles of the forearm. Stand in chest deep water with your arms bent at the elbow at a right angle. Keep the wrists in the water and hold the upper arms gently against your body with the elbows touching your sides. The palms of the hands should touch each other with the thumbs up towards the ceiling. The hands move up and down as the wrists are extended and flexed. (The elbows stay at a right angle.) You may exercise both wrists at the same time or can choose to alternate the wrists. This exercise should be repeated four to eight times.

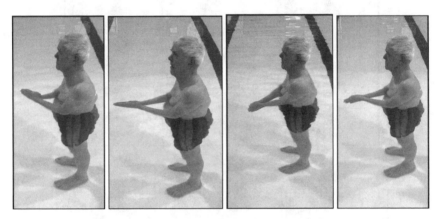

Figure 59: Wrist Flexion and Extension

Wrist Circles

Stand in chest deep water with your arms bent at the elbow at a right angle and rotate your hands at the wrist joint in a circular motion. Start by rotating both hands in towards the midline of the body with the right hand rotating in a counterclockwise circle and the left hand rotating in a clockwise circle. Repeat this movement six to eight times and then reverse the circles for six to eight times.

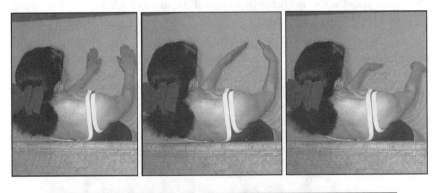

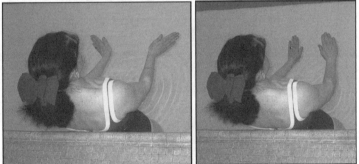

Figure 60: Wrist Circles

Fingers

It is important to warm up the joints of the fingers so they are ready to use pool equipment. The joints of the fingers are hinge joints with an ellipsoidal joint at the base of the finger. The ellipsoidal joint allows bending/extending with limited side-to-side movement. Stand in chest deep water with your arms bent at the elbow at a right angle. Try to touch each finger to the thumb to create an "O" shape. Start by touching the index finger tip to the thumb and end with the little finger. This is accomplished by placing the tip of each finger on the tip of the thumb. After completing each "O", the fingers should straighten to form a "V" shape. Repeat the sequence starting with the little finger and end with the index finger. Try to do two to four sequences with each hand.

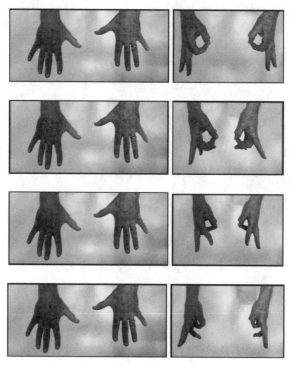

Figure 61: Fingers

Neck One

The neck flexibility exercises help to relieve stiffness and tension as well as helping to maintain flexibility in the joints and muscles of the neck. The joints of the neck are pivotal joints that allow you to turn your head from side to side or nod up and down. Hold your head upright so your chin is parallel to the pool floor. Keep your chin parallel to the pool floor and slowly turn the head to the right as much as is comfortable and pause. Then slowly turn the head to the left and pause. Repeat this motion six to eight times.

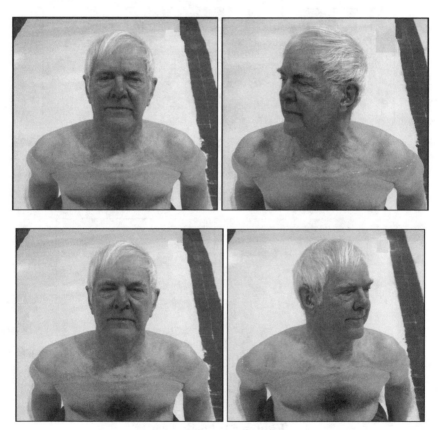

Figure 62: Neck One

Neck Two

Hold your head upright so the chin is parallel to the pool floor. Slowly drop the right ear toward the right shoulder and pause. Keeping the shoulders down and relaxed, bring the head slowly back to an upright position and then slowly drop the left ear toward the left shoulder and pause. It is important to keep the shoulders down and relaxed and avoid the urge to hunch the shoulders up so the ears touch the shoulders.

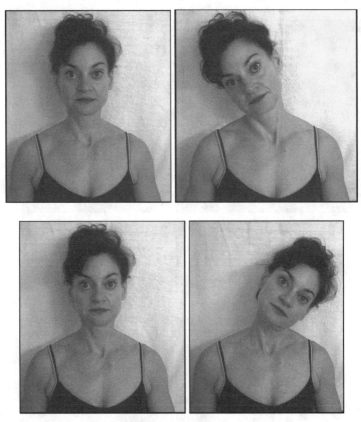

Figure 63: Neck Two

9

Stretches

Stretching is very important for people with rheumatoid arthritis. Stretching helps you to counter the stiffness caused by prolonged periods of sitting or inactivity. When you sit for long periods of time, your mobilizer muscles shorten. Stretching helps to lengthen the muscles and increase range of motion. Stretching should be done on a daily basis. Stretching in the water instead of on land may be more comfortable and easier for people who have difficulty with balance.

The stretches in this section give you numerous opportunities to vary your stretching workout. When choosing which stretches to do during a session, it is important to choose at least one stretch for each muscle or muscle group. A balance between agonist and antagonist muscles should be maintained.

How to Stretch

While stretching keep these ideas in mind:
- Move slowly and don't bounce. Moving slowly through a stretch overrides the reflex reaction and increases the elasticity of the muscles. Bouncing while stretching will cause the muscles to tighten instead of loosen and could result in a pulled muscle.
- Stretch to the point of mild muscle tension and not to the point of pain. Stretching beyond a mild tension can cause injury. Once

mild muscle tension has been reached, hold the stretch for 10 to 15 seconds.
* Breathe deeply with long inhalations and slow exhalations. Deep controlled breathing relaxes the muscles and brings them oxygen. This allows the muscle fibers to stretch more easily.

The stretches illustrated are for hips, calves, hamstrings, quadriceps, inner thigh, chest, triceps, wrists, and fingers.

Quadriceps Stretch One

This stretch targets the muscles located in the front of the thigh. Stand in waist to chest deep water with your side to the pool ledge. You may wish to use the pool ledge for support. Stand with your knees together and bring the right lower leg behind until the right ankle can be supported in your right hand. You need to keep the right knee pointing down to the pool floor and the back straight. To increase the stretch, push the right hip forward. During the stretch, you need to keep the thighs parallel and stationary. Hold the stretch for 10 to 15 seconds and then repeat with the right leg.

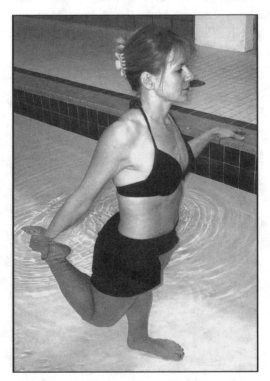

Figure 64: Quadriceps Stretch One

Quadriceps Stretch Two

This variation has a companion help you if you are not able to lift your leg very high or very well. The companion moves the leg into the stretching position. Working with a companion allows you to use both hands for support on the ledge of the pool.

Stand in waist to chest deep water facing the pool wall. The companion stands behind you and gently helps you bring your leg behind to a comfortable level while supporting the ankle. You and the companion will need to communicate so that the companion does not inadvertently pull the heel up too far or too fast. You will need to tell the companion when the stretch is at a comfortable tension and proper stretch resistance is reached. Hold the stretch for 10 to 15 seconds and repeat with the other leg. This is a good stretch for people who have balance problems.

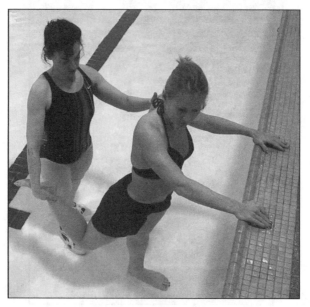

Figure 65: Quadriceps Stretch Two

Quadriceps Stretch Three

This is a good variation for people who have good balance but have limited flexibility in their thighs. In this modification, stand with your back to the pool stairs and place a hand on the pool ledge for added stability. Instead of lifting the heel up in back, place the top of your foot on one of the pool stairs and slowly lower yourself down towards the pool floor until a comfortable stretch is felt in the front of the thigh.

This stretch may also be done with the assistance of a companion. Stand with your back to the stairs and face the companion. Place your hands on the companion's shoulders and position the top of your foot on the stair. As you lower yourself down to facilitate the stretch, the companion helps keep you stable. Hold the stretch for 10 to 15 seconds and repeat with the other leg.

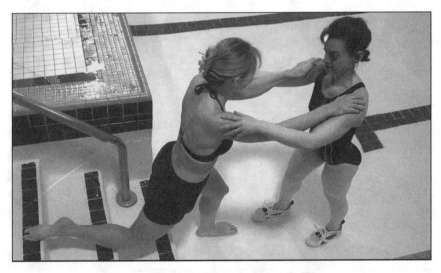

Figure 66: Quadriceps Stretch Three

Hamstring Stretch One

Stand in waist to chest deep water facing the pool wall. While standing at arm's length from the wall and holding the ledge for balance, place the right foot flat against the wall somewhere below the right hand. The foot should be placed so that only mild muscle tension is felt and not any pain. For some people the placement of the foot on the wall will be only a few inches from the pool floor, and for others the leg may be parallel with the pool floor. Regardless of where the foot is on the wall, as long as there is mild muscle tension, the stretch is working. During the stretch you must keep your back straight so the stretch is felt in the hamstring and not in the lower back. Hold the stretch for 10 to 15 seconds and then switch to the other leg.

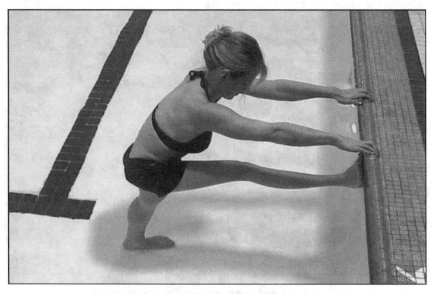

Figure 67: Hamstring Stretch One, one leg

An alternative is to place both feet on the wall in order to stretch the hamstrings of both legs at the same time.

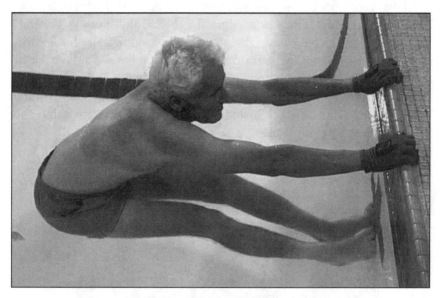

Figure 68: Hamstring Stretch One, two legs

Hamstring Stretch Two

This variation of the hamstring stretch is good for people who have trouble with balance or are less flexible. Hold onto the stair rail for support and prop your right heel up on a pool stair that is at a comfortable height so that a mild muscle tension is felt in the back of the thigh. While you are stretching, you will need to keep your back straight. Hold the stretch for 10 to 15 seconds and then repeat with the left leg. This is an active assisted stretch because you are using the stairs to assist with the stretch.

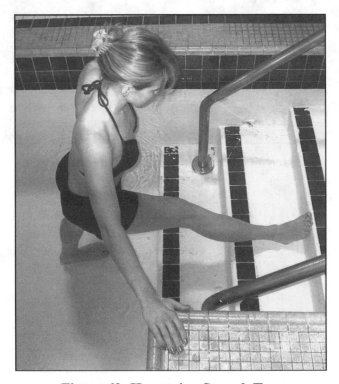

Figure 69: Hamstring Stretch Two

Calf Stretch

Stand in waist to chest deep water, an arm's length from the pool wall, do a pelvic tilt to insure good posture, bring the right foot back, and press the right heel down on the pool floor. If you are unable to reach the pool floor with the heel, you should try to bring the heel as close to the pool floor as is comfortable. To increase the stretch, bend the arms at the elbows and lean toward the pool wall. Hold the stretch for 10 to 15 seconds and repeat with the other leg.

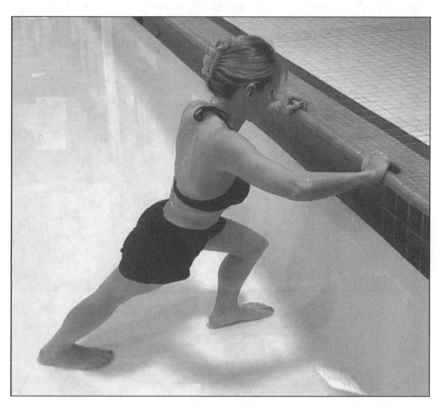

Figure 70: Calf Stretch

Inner Thigh Stretch

This stretch will make it much easier to climb stairs, get into buses or subways, and walk. This stretch also helps to lengthen the stride. In water that is waist to chest deep, stand facing the pool wall, an arm's length from the ledge. Placing the feet apart and facing the hips toward the wall, bend the right leg slightly, making sure the knee does not extend as far as the toes. It is important for you to keep the left leg straight, but not locked at the knee, and to keep the foot flat on the floor. The stretch can be increased by starting with the feet wider apart or by bending the knee of the non-stretching leg a little more. Hold the stretch for 10 to 15 seconds and repeat with the other leg.

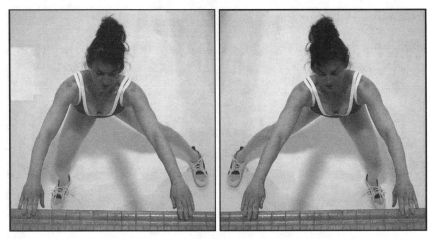

Figure 71: Inner Thigh Stretch

Hips Stretch One

Stand in waist to chest deep water, an arm's length from the pool wall. Using the pool wall for support, stand tall, with legs hip's width apart and the left leg back behind with the heel resting on or close to the pool floor. The toes of both feet should be facing forward with the buttocks tucked under the hips. The hips should be rotated forward and up and the left knee should be slightly bent. This movement will cause a stretching sensation that will be felt in the front of the hip of the leg that is back. Hold this stretch for 10 to 15 seconds and then stretch the other side.

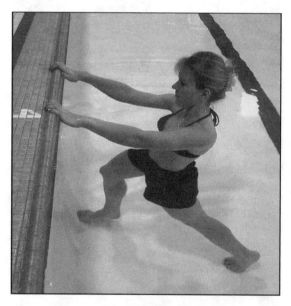

Figure 72: Hips Stretch One

Hips Stretch Two

This stretch keeps the hip flexor (the muscle that extends from the outer hip down to the inside knee) supple. Stand in waist to chest deep water and use the pool ledge for support with one or two hands as shown in the pictures. Place the right foot one step behind the left leg and as far to the left as is comfortable. Then with both feet flat on the floor, lean the right hip farther toward the right. Hold the stretch for 10 to 15 seconds and then repeat with the other hip.

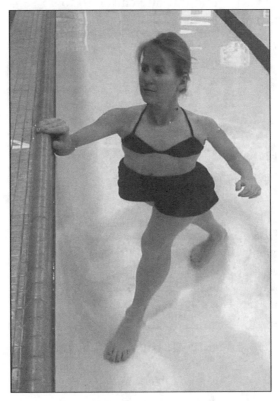

Figure 73: Hips Stretch Two, front view

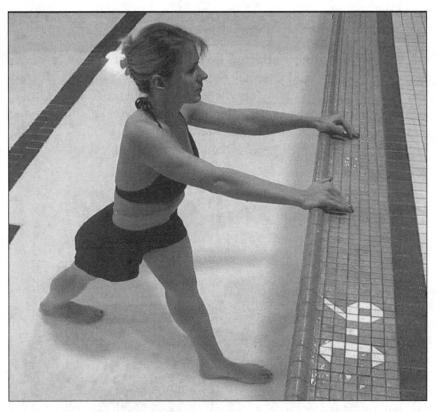

Figure 74: Hips Stretch Two, side view

Side Stretch

The muscle groups affected by this stretch are the sides of the torso (the internal and external obliques) and the back (specifically the erector spinae). Stand in chest deep water with the feet hip's width apart. Reach over your head with the right arm without shifting your hips. This movement causes the stretch to be felt on the right side. Hold the stretch for 10 to 15 seconds and then repeat on the other side.

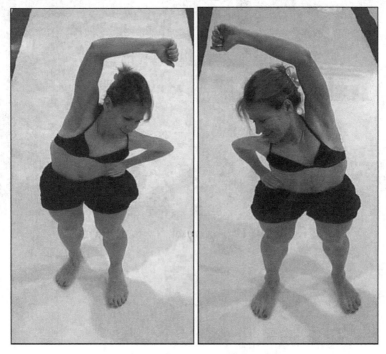

Figure 75: Side Stretch, done alone

If you have limited flexibility, a companion may assist you by placing a hand around your waist and gently guiding the arm into the proper position. The companion needs to be careful not to extend the stretch too far.

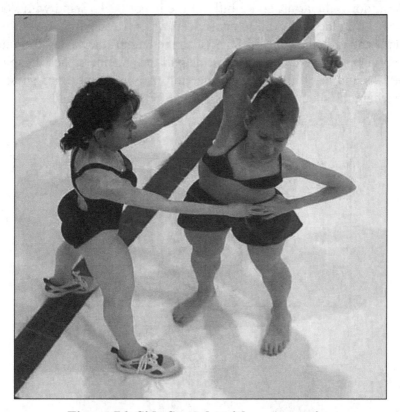

Figure 76: Side Stretch, with a companion

Chest Stretch One

This stretch is good for offsetting curved and rounded shoulders and for improving breathing. The stretch should be felt across the chest, down the arms, and a little in the upper back. Stand with your back facing the pool wall in chest deep water. Reach around with the hands and grab the edge of the pool so the thumbs face away from the body. Lean forward and let the arms pull the shoulders back, keeping the ribs and head lifted up and the chin parallel to the floor without hunching the shoulders. Hold the stretch for 10 to 15 seconds.

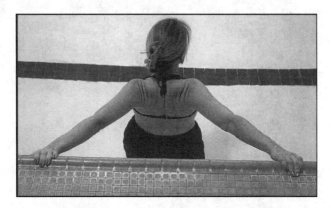

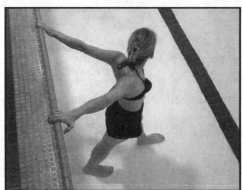

Figure 77: Chest Stretch One, back view and side view

Chest Stretch Two

You and the companion stand in chest deep water with the companion standing behind you. Extend your arms behind your back. The companion gently supports your hands by having you place your hands in the companion's palms. As you lean forward and lengthen your arms, the companion can gently interlock his or her fingers with your fingers for support. Hold the stretch for 10 to 15 seconds. This is an especially good variation if you have trouble gripping the ledge of the pool.

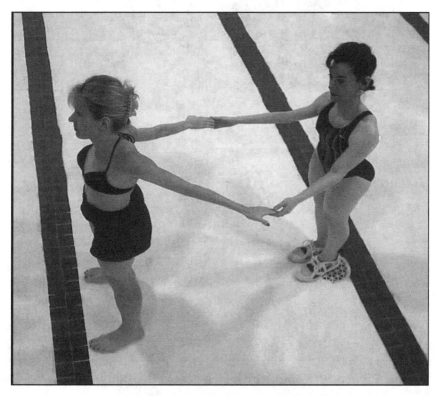

Figure 78: Chest Stretch Two

Shoulder Stretch across the Body

This stretch is good for loosening up the back of the arms and the shoulders. Stand in waist to chest deep water. Bring your right arm across the front of your chest and grasp the lower arm with the left hand. It is important that you do not grab the elbow joint. Gently guide the arm across the chest and hold the stretch for 15 to 20 seconds. Relax and repeat the stretch with the other arm.

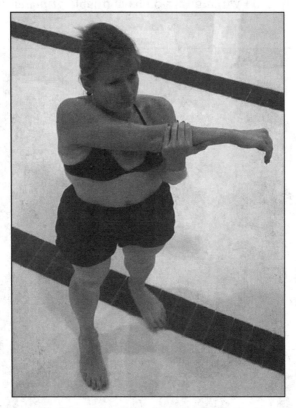

Figure 79: Shoulder Stretch across the Body, alone

If you have limited mobility, a companion can assist by placing a hand on the shoulder for added stability. Once you are comfortable, the companion guides your arm across your body. Make sure you stand straight and tall without twisting at the waist.

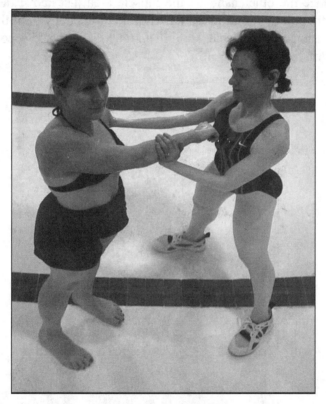

Figure 80: Shoulder Stretch across the Body, with a companion

Triceps Stretch

This stretch loosens the muscles located at the back of the upper arm. Standing in chest deep water, raise your right arm over your head. Place the other hand on the muscle area just above the elbow and gently pull the arm toward the midline of the body until there is a slight tension in the muscle. Hold the stretch for 10 to 15 seconds and repeat with the other arm.

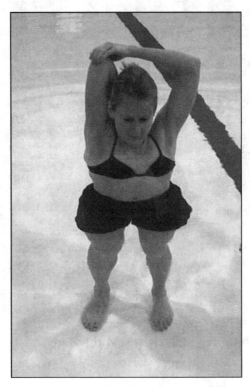

Figure 81: Triceps Stretch, alone

A companion may offer assistance if you are not flexible enough to fully accomplish this stretch. The companion can help guide your arm into the proper position and support the arm just above the elbow joint. Hold the stretch for 10 to 15 seconds and then repeat with the other arm.

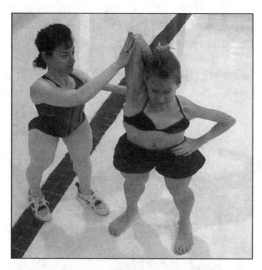

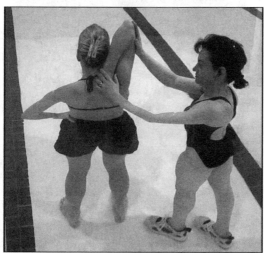

Figure 82: Triceps Stretch, with a companion

Fingers Stretch One

This movement helps to prevent the fingers from curling in. While in the water, place your hands just below the surface of the water and spread the fingers of one hand out wide and flat as if to span a great distance. Hold this position for a count of ten and rest. You may alternate by stretching one hand at a time or you may stretch both hands at the same time.

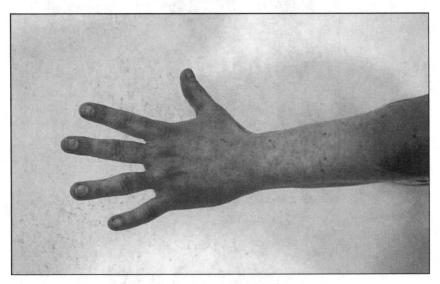

Figure 83: Fingers Stretch One

Fingers Stretch Two

Spread the fingers of the left hand out and press the palm of the right hand under the fingers of the left hand making sure to avoid the fingertips. Then press slightly on the outspread hand and hold for a count of ten before taking a small break. Repeat the sequence with the other hand.

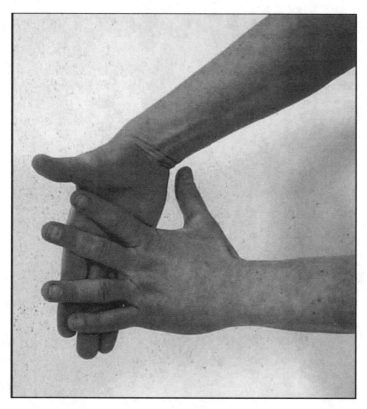

Figure 84: Fingers Stretch Two

10

Aerobic Exercises

Aerobic exercises increase the amount of oxygen used by the body and help to condition the heart, lungs, and circulatory system. They are also called endurance, cardiovascular, or cardio-respiratory exercises. The goal of an aerobic exercise is to reach your target heart rate and hold it there for at least 15 to 20 minutes. To be truly aerobic, the exercises must be done nonstop for an extended period of time. It is the sustained exercise that helps increase aerobic fitness.

To reach the target heart rate requires doing some relatively energetic exercise with the large muscle groups. The primary muscles used in these aerobic exercises are the buttocks, thighs, and calves.

Warm-up exercises can be expanded into aerobic exercises by increasing their duration (and perhaps their intensity). For example, the Water Cycle and the Water Jog are good warm-ups when done for three to five minutes but become aerobic when done for 15 minutes or longer. Aerobic exercises should not be done to the point of exhaustion. You should be able to breathe easily and carry on a light conversation while exercising. If you become too winded to speak in complete sentences, then the intensity of the exercise needs to be reduced.

The aerobic pace will vary with your condition and experience. In the beginning you will need to start at a slow pace and gradually build up. It might even mean starting with five minutes and working up to 20 to 30 minutes over the course of a few weeks. The more conditioned and experienced you become, the longer and more vigorous the aerobics portion can be. No matter what level of ability you have, you should always be aware of pain, flare-ups, and swelling in the joints and muscles and not exercise under these conditions.

To vary the aerobic routine, you can choose to do a number of different types of aerobic moves or you may choose to do one move for an extended period of time. If the aerobic workout is divided among different exercises, you should make sure the transitions between the exercises are short so the aerobic benefits of the exercise are not lost

If you have rheumatoid arthritis or if you are experiencing joint swelling, you may wish to perform the Cross Country Ski as a low impact exercise because the drag force offers strength training in the form of resistance and yet does not place undue stress on the joints.

Straight Leg Aerobic Kick

This exercise uses the large muscles of the hips, buttocks, and thighs and helps with balance as well as aerobic conditioning. Standing tall with a neutral spine, contracted abdominal muscles, and with your side to the pool wall, do a leg kick. This motion is similar to marchers performing the "goose step." At the same time, swing the arm that is on the same side forward from the shoulder with the palm facing up. Then alternate these leg and arm motions with enough force and speed to be challenging but not exhausting. If you feel unsteady when incorporating the arms, you may omit them until you feel steadier and even use the pool ledge for support. You can intensify the exercise by increasing the number of leg lifts per minute, increasing the duration of the exercise, and/or incorporating the property of drag by moving through the water.

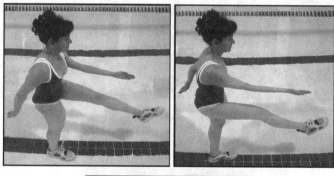

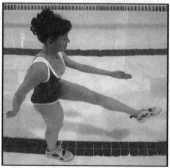

Figure 85: Straight Leg Aerobic Kick

Knee Lifts

Stand in waist to chest deep water with your side to the pool wall. As you move through the water, lift your knees in an alternating fashion as if marching, raising the thigh so it is parallel to the pool floor. The opposite arm is lifted from the shoulder with the palms up. This exercise helps to lubricate the hip and knee joints as well as promoting balance.

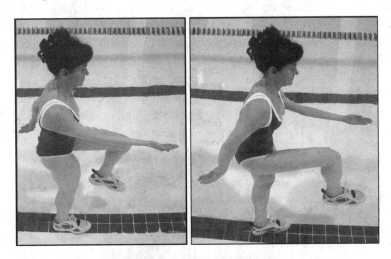

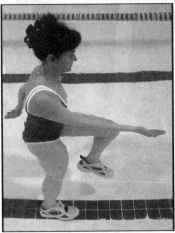

Figure 86: Knee Lifts

You may wish to work with a partner or trainer. The partner can walk along side of you to help with balance and extend a hand forward at hip level as a guide for your knee. This will encourage you to lift your knee to the proper height.

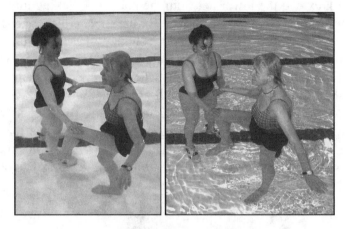

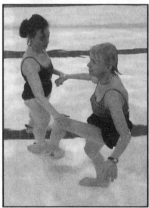

Figure 87: Knee Lifts with a partner

Knee Lift with Leg Extension

In this exercise, you are in waist to chest deep water with your side to the pool wall. Once the knee is lifted (as in the Knee Lift exercise), extend the lower leg from the knee in a kicking motion and then bring the straight leg down to the pool floor. Repeat the movement with the other leg and continue these motions in an alternating fashion. The arms are lifted from the shoulder with the palms facing upward. Lift one arm when the knee goes up. Switch arms when the leg extends. Put both arms back down when the leg goes down. This is another exercise that promotes balance as well as coordination. If a trainer is working with you, he or she may walk alongside you using an extended hand as a guide for your knee and also moving a hand along the leg as a guide for the leg extension.

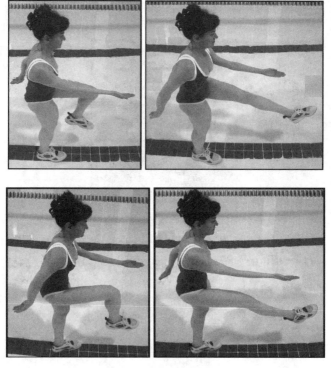

Figure 88: Knee Lifts with Leg Extension

Cross Country Ski

This is a great aerobic exercise because it uses muscles from both the lower body and the upper body. In chest deep water, arm's length from the pool wall, shift your weight from one leg to the other as you move through the water. It is important to keep a slight bend in the knee that is bearing your weight. As the right leg is brought forward, swing the right arm forward from the shoulder with a cupped, forward-facing hand. As you pull the leg behind, the hand is shifted to a backward-facing position in order to continue grabbing water. This allows you to take advantage of the water's resistance. The arms and legs are moved in a skiing motion. You may wish to use water gloves for extra resistance.

If it is not too stressful to your hip and knee joints, a slight bounce may be added to the skiing motion in order to add more intensity to the exercise.

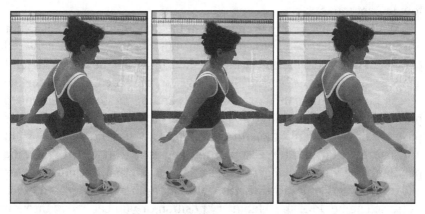

Figure 89: Cross Country Ski

Pendulum Swing

In this exercise the lower body and the upper body are being used together with the core as an articulation point, which helps to enhance your sense of balance and coordination. Stand in chest deep water, arm's length from the pool ledge, facing the pool wall. In an alternating fashion, shift your weight from one foot to the other in a side-to-side pendulum motion. Start with all of your weight on the right leg and lift the left leg out to the side from the hip joint as high up as possible. Then hop on the right foot to return the left foot to the pool floor. The right leg is lifted up as high as possible to the right. Then hop on the left foot to bring the right leg down and the left leg up again and so on in a pendulum swing. The hydrostatic pressure of the water at chest deep level should provide enough cushioning for the hip, knee, and ankle joints, but if there is pain in the joints, the hop can be eliminated and the pendulum movement can be modified to a low impact move.

While the lower body is engaged in the pendulum swing, use your arms to push the water down. When your body weight is centered over the right foot, the left arm is pulled up from the shoulder joint and the lower arm is bent at the elbows so the forearm is under the biceps muscle. The palms of your hands are facing down in a cupped position. As you are ready to alternate to the left leg, the left arm is pushed downward until the arm is straight. At the same time, the right arm is drawn up to the ready position and is then released when the pendulum swing is changed. Both of these alternating motions flex and extend the oblique muscles, thus strengthening the core. This exercise can be done in a stationary position or you can move through the water. You can make the exercise more intense by shortening the time between the alternating moves as you move forward and backward.

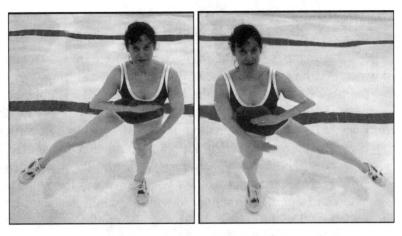

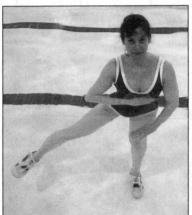

Figure 90: Pendulum Swing

The Water Jog

The Water Jog uses the large muscles of the legs. In waist to chest deep water, standing tall with a neutral spine, alternate lifting your leg up off the pool floor, bending at the knee, and kicking back the heel. You may want to stand arm's length from the pool wall in case the ledge is needed for support. Standing in chest deep water offers more cushioning effect for the knee and hip joints compared to standing in waist deep water. The faster you alternate your feet, the more intense the exercise becomes. Another way for you to intensify the Water Jog is to move while jogging (from one side of the pool to the other, laps, or in a circle). The movement causes a drag effect, which adds resistance to the exercise. If you are in chest deep water and are jogging at a good pace, drag will make the exercise more intense than in waist deep water.

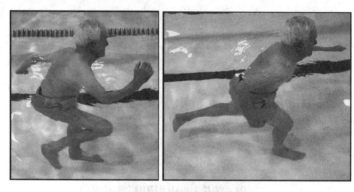

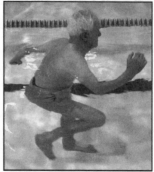

Figure 91: The Water Jog

Water Run with Swinging Arms

This aerobic exercise is identical to the Water Walk featured in the warm-up section, but instead of walking, run in place or, for a more intense aerobic workout, run through the water. Running involves lifting the legs higher and faster than walking. When running, you will push yourself off of the pool floor with one foot and be suspended momentarily until you land on the other foot. While running, move your arms from the shoulders back and forth with the arms bent at an angle at the elbows. If the joints are too uncomfortable to sustain a running movement, you may walk as fast as possible to achieve aerobic benefits.

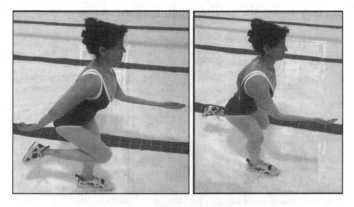

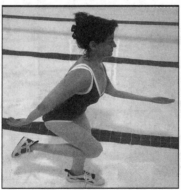

Figure 92: Water Run with Swinging Arms

Water Run with Breast Stroke Arms

Stand in chest deep water and run back and forth or in a small circle. At the same time bring your hands close to your chest with elbows out to the side and the palms of the hands close together. As you run or jog through the water, push your hands forward, rotating them at the wrist so the palms face outward and attempt to part the water in a breaststroke. The stroke is completed when the arms circle around and are brought back to the starting position. This aerobic exercise can be done with the assistance of a companion and you may want to stay close to the pool edge for balance. This Water Run is a more intense version of the Water Walk with Breast Stroke Arms. For a full aerobic effect, this exercise should alternate with other aerobic exercises such as the Water Run with Rowing Arms.

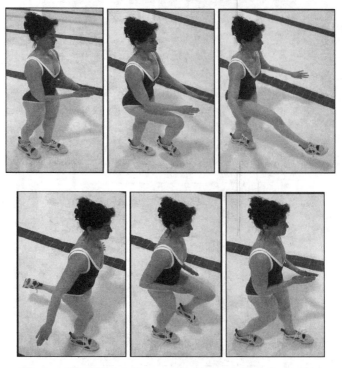

Figure 93: Water Run with Breast Stroke Arms

Water Run with Rowing Arms

Stand in chest deep water and run back and forth or in a small circle. Start with your arms outstretched at the sides and just under the water surface. As you run, the arms swing around to the front and scoop water with the palms of the hands and then the arms fold in at the elbows and the hands fold in at the wrist as the arms come towards the chest. Your fingers then follow the line of your arms as the arms open up to begin again. For a full aerobic effect, this exercise should alternate with other aerobic exercises for a period of at least 15 minutes.

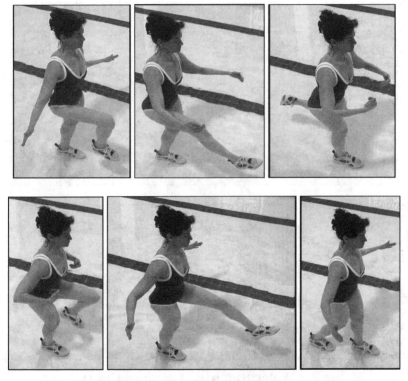

Figure 94: Water Run with Rowing Arms

Water Run with American Crawl

Stand in chest deep water close enough to the pool wall for comfort and support. As you run or jog through the water, rotate the arms from the shoulders as if doing the American crawl swimming stroke. To start, the arms are extended out front with the palms facing down. As you run, the right arm swings down from the shoulder and reaches as far back as is comfortable. The palm is then turned up and the arm is brought up out of the water and then with the palm rotated down, the arm is returned to the water. The left arm makes the same kind of circle, starting when the right arm comes out of the water. The alternating circle pattern continues as you run or jog continuously.

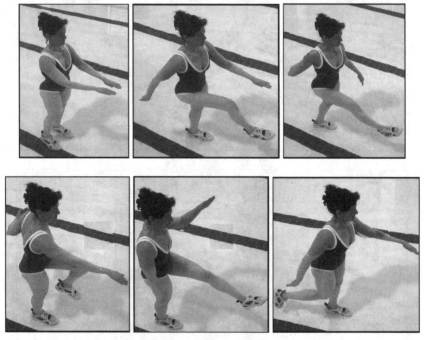

Figure 95: Water Run with American Crawl Arms

Rocking Horse with Push-Pull Arms

Stand in waist to chest deep water a comfortable distance from the pool wall. Bring your left knee up to chest level and balance on the right foot. Bending the arms slightly at the elbows, bring the arms and hands up just under the surface of the water. The palms of the hands are up and in a cupped position. Then rock forward so the left foot is planted on the pool floor. As the left foot comes down, the right leg is brought up in back with a bent knee. Extend the arms with the hands open and flat so they can push the water down in front. Then step up with the right foot to where the left foot landed and raise the left knee again. Continue this rocking motion through the water or in a circle. After rocking about 30 feet, switch legs so the right leg is in front and the left leg rocks back. Switch which leg is in front every 30 feet or so. You may wish to use a long bar bell or water gloves for added resistance when pushing and pulling against the water.

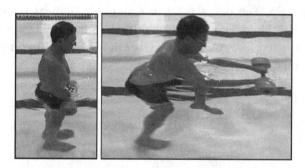

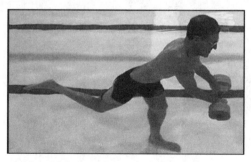

Figure 96: Rocking Horse with Push-Pull Arms using a Barbell

Exercises Using the Water Jogging Belt

Water jogging belts are especially good for people who have arthritis because the hips, knees, and feet may be sensitive to the impact of landing on the pool floor. Exercises done while wearing a water jogging belt need to be performed in water deep enough to suspend you off the pool bottom.

The exercises performed with the water jogging belt are The Water Jog, Cross Country Ski, Straight Leg Scissor Cross, Flutter Kicks, Treading Water, Single Leg Circles (done from the hip), Double Leg Circles (done from the hip), and the Bicycle. Some of these exercises can also be performed in the pool as aerobic exercises without a jogging belt.

You need to put the jogging belt on before you enter the pool. Most jogging belts have Velcro closures or big clips as fasteners. However, if you have trouble with your hands, a companion or fitness trainer can help. The belt should fit snuggly but not be so tight that it constricts breathing. The jogging belt is designed to keep you upright at all times. Therefore, under no circumstances should you try to do a flip or a somersault while wearing the jogging belt.

Water Jog Using the Jogging Belt

The Water Jog Using the Jogging Belt is similar to the Water Jog in the previous section. Put the jogging belt on before entering the water. Once in the water, stand tall with a neutral spine in water that is deep enough for your feet to be suspended off the bottom of the pool. You may wish to remain arm's length from the pool wall for safety reasons. Alternate lifting your leg up toward the chest, bending at the knee, and kicking the heel back. The faster you move, the more intense the exercise becomes. You may jog in one place or jog in a circle for a few minutes and then reverse the circle. As long as you are in deep enough water, you may move forward or backward in a straight line.

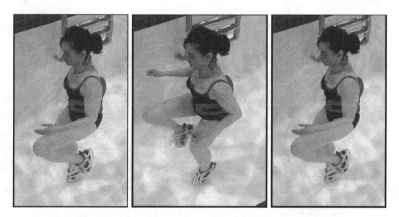

Figure 97: Water Jog Using the Jogging Belt

Cross Country Ski Using the Jogging Belt

Wearing a jogging belt in water that is deep enough so your feet are not touching the pool floor, move your legs forward and backward from the hip joint with relaxed feet. The legs remain straight. The arms move forward and backward from the shoulders in a scissor-type movement so one arm is lifted forward and the other arm is pulling backward. The right arm goes forward with the left foot and vice versa. The palms of the hands should face the direction the arms are moving, cupping the water to gain the benefits of the water's resistance. Water gloves can be used to increase the resistance. You need to remain an arm's length from the pool ledge so you can maneuver yourself to shallower water in order to exit the pool when you are done.

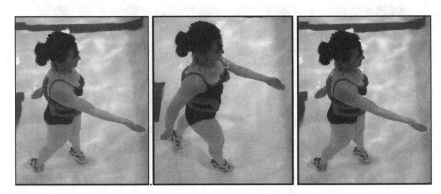

Figure 98: Cross Country Ski Using the Jogging Belt

Straight Leg Scissor Cross

This exercise is done in the frontal plane and exercises the leg adductors/abductors and the gluteus. Wear a jogging belt in water deep enough to suspend yourself off the pool floor. Start with the legs straight and just beyond shoulder width apart. Then bring the legs together, crossing at the ankles. Spreads the legs back apart and bring them together crossing at the ankles once again. When crossing at the ankles, alternate having the right and left ankle in front. The faster the legs are moved, the more drag and resistance you will generate.

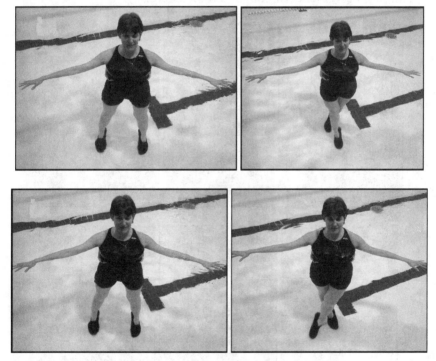

Figure 99: Straight Leg Scissor Cross

Flutter Kicks

Wear a jogging belt in water deep enough to suspend yourself off the pool floor an arm's length from the pool ledge. With legs straight and close together, alternate kicking your legs in short, tight rapid crisscross motions from the hips. The right and left foot take turns being in front. The Flutter Kick is a very intense move. When doing the Flutter Kick, you will notice your heart rate increasing. The Flutter Kick is very good for cardiovascular training since it can be used as an interval training exercise and can be mixed in as an alternating movement with other aerobic exercises.

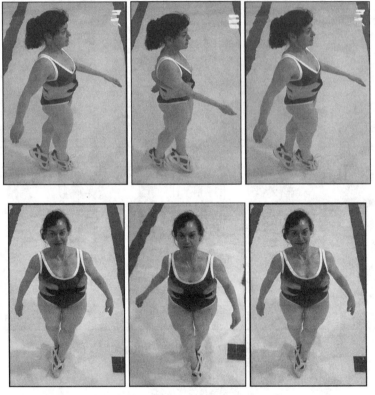

Figure 100: Flutter Kicks, side and front views

An example of using the Flutter Kick intermittently with another aerobic exercise is to combine the Straight Leg Scissor Cross and Flutter Kick into one aerobic workout. Start with a Scissor Kick for two to three minutes and then do a Flutter Kick for 15 to 30 seconds and then return to the Scissor Kick for two to three minutes and then do a Flutter kick for another 15 to 30 seconds. Try to alternate this pattern for five to ten minutes and then proceed to another aerobic exercise.

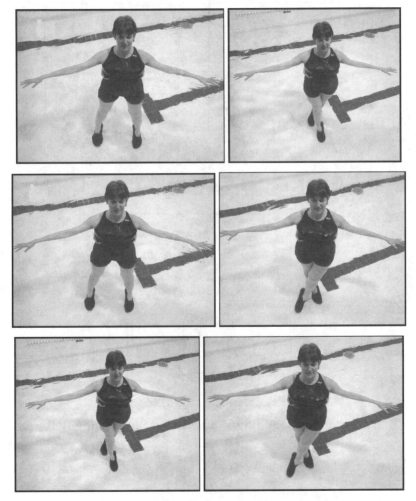

Figure 101: Scissor Cross and Flutter Kicks

Treading Water Using the Jogging Belt

Float in water deep enough to be suspended off the pool bottom, an arm's length from the wall. With relaxed hips, knees, ankles, and feet, move the legs back and forth in a rhythmic, steady motion. This is a very good endurance exercise since it can be done for a very long time at a very steady level.

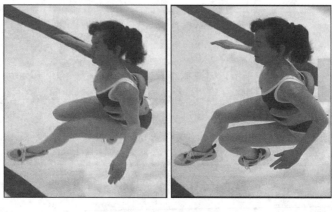

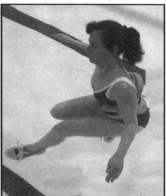

Figure 102: Treading Water Using the Jogging Belt

Single Leg Circle Using the Jogging Belt

Wear a jogging belt in water deep enough so you are off the pool floor. You may wish to use the pool ledge for support. With the right side closest to the pool wall, circle your left leg from the hip rotating clockwise, keeping the leg straight. Circle the leg for ten repetitions and then reverse the motion and rotate the leg counterclockwise for ten more repetitions. Then turn your body to the left side and repeat the circle motions with the right leg. Try to circle each leg clockwise and counterclockwise three to five times.

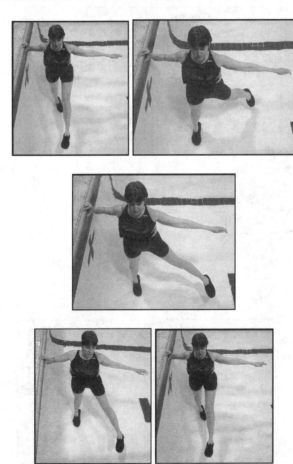

Figure 103: Single Leg Circle Using the Jogging Belt

Double Leg Circle Using the Jogging Belt

Wear a jogging belt in water deep enough so you are off the pool floor close to the pool wall. With your legs held close together rotate your legs from the hip in a circle going in a clockwise direction for 10 to 15 rotations and then switch the circle to a counterclockwise direction for 10 to 15 rotations. Try to do three to five sets of clockwise/counterclockwise rotations. The less time taken in changing direction, the more drag effect and aerobic benefits you will experience.

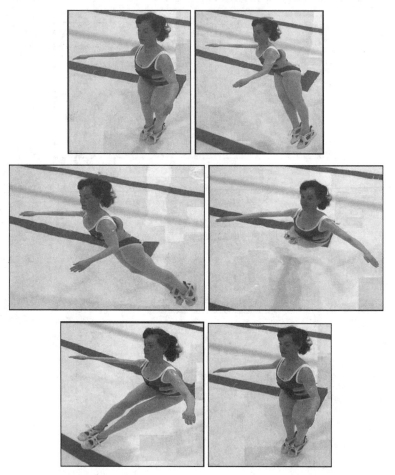

Figure 104: Double Leg Circle Using the Jogging Belt

Bicycle Using the Jogging Belt

Wear a jogging belt in water deep enough so you are off the pool floor an arm's length from the pool ledge. Circle the legs forward and backwards in an alternating motion and alternate bending the legs at the knee joint and straightening the leg. The motion should mimic the action of riding a bicycle. The motion should be rhythmic, smooth, and steady and can be done for a long time. This is another very good long endurance exercise.

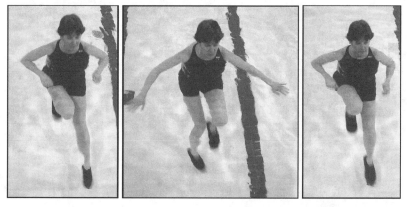

Figure 105: Bicycle Using the Jogging Belt

11

Strength Training Exercises

Strength training, resistance training, and weight lifting all refer to exercises that build muscle. Strength training helps to build muscle that supports the joints that bear the load of your weight. Well supported joints are less painful and more efficient, making movement easier. Muscle strength can be built and maintained with regular weight lifting.

For people with rheumatoid arthritis, lifting weights on land can cause pain because gravity puts more pressure on the joints. Using weights that are designed to be used in the water or just using the water's resistance alone can replace using heavy weights on land. The water cushions the joints through hydrostatic pressure and helps to support the joints while the water's resistance strengthens the muscles.

Strength training exercises involve the use of long lever moves and short lever moves. Long lever moves use the entire arm or leg as a straight lever and the movement points are located at the shoulder and the hip. Long lever moves can be performed in the frontal, sagittal, and transverse planes because the shoulder and hip joints are ball and socket joints and allow movement in all directions. Short lever moves use half of the arm or half of the leg. The articulation points are the elbow and knee, which are hinge joints. Hinge joints can move either up and down or side to side. Gliding joints are a combination of two hinge joints and are found in the wrists and ankles.

Many of the strength training exercises are adapted from the warm-up exercises with the addition of water weights, bar bells, dumbbells, kick boards, noodles, and water gloves. There are strength-training exercises for upper body, lower body, and the torso.

As you are doing the strength training exercises, remember to work the muscles in an agonist-antagonist pair. For example, if you exercise the quadriceps on the front of the leg, be sure to exercise the hamstrings on the back of the leg to keep them in balance. Strength is important, but balanced muscle pairs are even more important for healthy movement.

Water is a great place to do strength training because it is very hard to get unbalanced muscles. If you look at the Leg Lift Front and the Leg Pull, you will see that both exercises use the same movement. The only difference is that one makes the forceful movement up and the other makes the forceful movement down. When you exercise in the water, all of your muscles are getting a workout, even when you are concentrating especially hard on one of them.

Lower Body Strength Training, Long Lever

Long lever exercises for the lower body involve the hip joint, which is a ball and socket joint. This allows exercises to be performed in all the different planes. Movement can be up and down, side-to-side, or rotational. The articulation point is the hip. Long lever exercises can be performed in more than one plane at a time. The hip joint is involved in activities such as getting in and out of cars, chairs, and bathtubs. The hip is also involved in walking, climbing, sitting, bending, and putting on clothes. Hips that work well make life much easier.

Leg Lift Front

This exercise strengthens the quadriceps. Stand in waist to chest deep water with your left side to the pool wall and with your arm on the pool ledge for support. Keeping the leg straight, the knee soft, and the foot relaxed, lift the right leg up in front and then return the leg to the starting position. Start with eight to ten repetitions and then relax for a few seconds before resuming another set of eight to ten repetitions. Take small breaks between sets. Then turn the body around so your right side is toward the pool wall and repeat the exercise with the left leg. It is advisable to start with a bare leg and then, when you feel strong enough, try to add ankle weights, water wings, or a noodle.

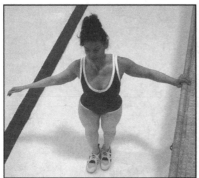 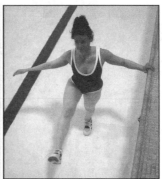

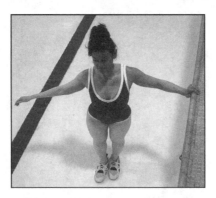

Figure 106: Leg Lift Front

Leg Pull

This exercise strengthens the hamstrings and the gluteus. Stand in waist to chest deep water with your side near the wall. Shift the body's weight to the left leg and extend the right leg out front from the hip. Keeping the leg straight, soft at the knee, and the foot relaxed, pull the right leg down until it is next to the left leg. Then lift the leg up again and then pull the leg down. As the leg is pulled down, contract the muscles of the hamstring and the gluteus. Start with eight to ten repetitions and take a few seconds to relax before doing eight to ten more until three sets are completed. Then shift your weight to the right leg and repeat the procedure with the left leg being sure to relax between sets. Once you feel strong enough, a noodle or ankle weights may be used for added resistance.

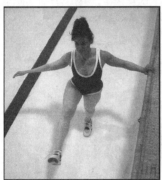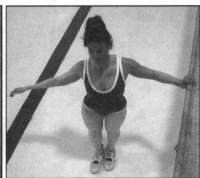

Figure 107: Leg Pull

Leg Swing

This exercise strengthens the quadriceps, the hamstrings, and the gluteus maximus and helps to keep the hip flexor supple. Stand in waist to chest deep water with your left side to the pool wall and your arm on the pool ledge for support. Starting with legs together and parallel, lift the right leg up in front keeping the leg straight, the knee soft, and the foot relaxed. Then in a controlled move, swing the right leg behind, as far back as possible, until contractions are felt in the buttocks and down the hamstring. The foot movement should be a vertical arc. As the foot comes close to the bottom of the pool floor, you will need to flex the foot so it does not touch the pool floor. Start with eight to ten arcs and then relax for a few seconds before repeating the set one or two more times. Then turn around and repeat the exercise with the left leg. Once you are proficient with this exercise you may wish to try it with water weights.

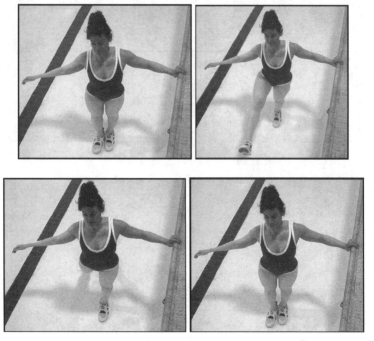

Figure 108: Leg Swing

Leg Lift Behind

The Leg Lift Behind strengthens the gluteus and the hamstrings. Stand with your side to the pool wall or face the pool wall. Either way, stand in waist to chest deep water using the pool wall for support. Starting with the legs parallel to each other, lift the right leg back until there is a contraction felt in the gluteus and hamstring and then bring the leg back to the parallel position. Keeping the knee soft and the foot relaxed start with eight to ten repetitions and continue to do three sets of eight to ten repetitions while taking a few seconds between sets to rest. Once you are proficient with this exercise, you may wish to try ankle weights.

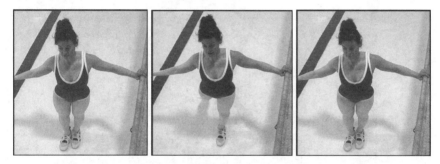

Figure 109: Leg Lift Behind, front view

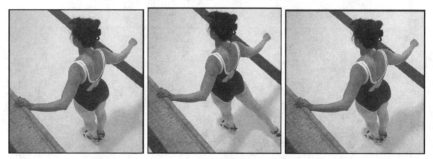

Figure 110: Leg Lift Behind, back view

Leg Circle

This exercise helps keep the hip joint supple as well as strengthening the muscles of the front, inner, back, and outer thigh. Stand with your right side to the pool wall in waist to chest deep water with your arm on the pool ledge for support. Raise the left leg forward at a 45° angle and circle the leg in a clockwise rotation keeping the knee soft and the foot relaxed. Then reverse the rotation so it is counterclockwise. It is important for you to keep the leg in the front and back plane and not to cross the midline. Start with eight to ten clockwise/counterclockwise circles and then rest. Try to do three sets of eight to ten on each leg. Leg weights can be added later.

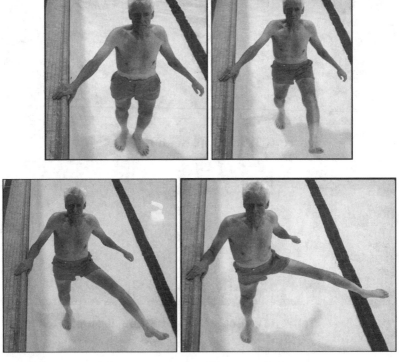

Figure 111: Leg Circle, starting

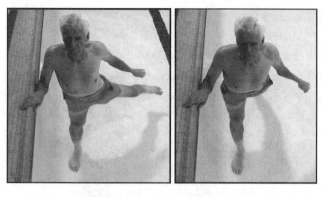

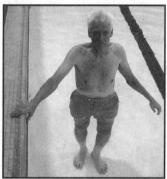

Figure 112: Leg Circle, finishing

Scissors

This exercise strengthens the inner and outer thighs. You are positioned in waist to chest deep water. You can have a noodle wrapped around your upper back, you can wear a jogging belt, or you can hold onto the pool ledge with your back against the pool wall if long as your shoulders and arms can support you. Your legs are parallel to the pool floor and extend straight out from the hip with the knees soft and the feet relaxed. Start with the legs slightly crossed, swing the legs apart, and then bring the legs together as if making the lower half of a snow angel. Start with two to three sets of eight to ten repetitions with a few seconds rest between each set. Water weights can be used for additional resistance.

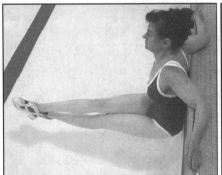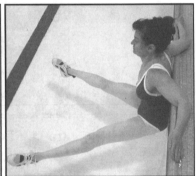

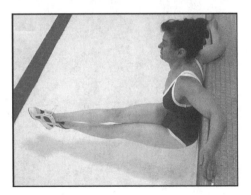

Figure 113: Scissors, using the wall

Side Leg Raises

This exercise strengthens the hip, adductor/abductors, back, and the buttocks and is done in the sagittal plane. Stand in water that is waist to chest deep with feet together and your right side to the pool wall. The right arm is on the pool ledge for support. Lift the left leg out to the side, keeping the leg straight with a soft knee and the toes facing forward and then return the leg to the starting position. Start with six to ten repetitions and then rest for a few seconds before doing two to three sets with rests between the sets. For added resistance ankle weights or a noodle may be used.

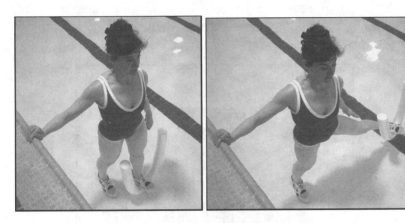

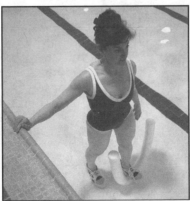

Figure 114: Side Leg Raises, using a noodle

Straight Leg Kicks

This exercise strengthens the front and back of the thighs and is done in a prone position using a kickboard or the ledge of the pool for support. Gently kick the water with a straight leg, moving from the hips and keeping the knee joint soft. This exercise does not need to be done in a stationary position. If you are using a kickboard, you may kick down the length of the pool and do laps. If you have trouble keeping your head held up because of limited mobility in the neck or arthritis in the spine, you may lie in a supine position using a noodle wrapped around your midsection for support. One kick with each leg is one repetition. Start with 10 to 15 repetitions and then relax for a few seconds before doing two to three sets with 10 to 15 repetitions in each set. Rest between the sets.

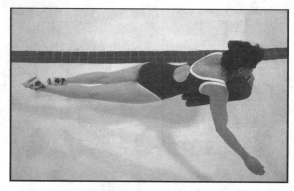

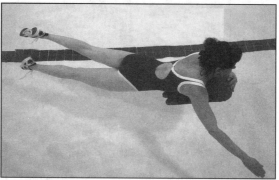

Figure 115: Straight Leg Kicks, using a kickboard in a prone position

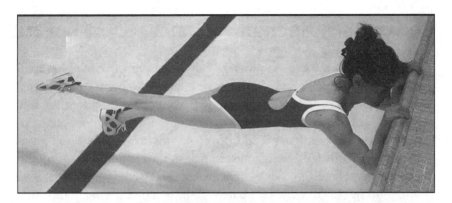

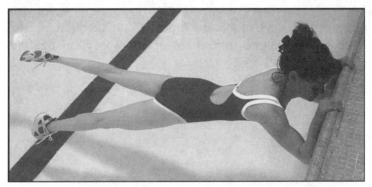

Figure 116: Straight Leg Kicks, off the wall

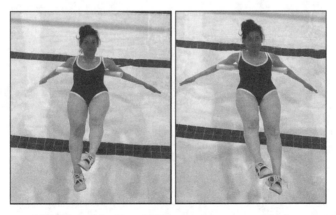

Figure 117: Straight Leg Kicks, using a noodle in a supine position

Lower Body Strength Training, Short Lever

Short lever moves for the lower body use a portion of the leg with the articulation point being the knee or ankle, which are hinge joints. As mentioned earlier, the ankle actually is a pair of hinge joints, one on top of the other, which allows bending in multiple directions. Hinge joints move either up and down or side to side. A hinge joint works one specific muscle or muscle pair at a time and only works in one plane at a time. Activities that involve the knee joint are sitting down, getting out of a chair or car, walking, and climbing. The ankle joint can work in more than one plane and is used for walking, driving, standing, and climbing. Since the ankle joint is a gliding joint, the proprioceptors in the ankle are especially important for balance.

Quadriceps

This exercise strengthens the front of the thigh. Stand with your back against the wall in waist to chest deep water. Shift your weight to the left leg and lift the right leg up at the hip bending at the knee. Keeping the thigh parallel to the pool floor, extend the lower leg out in front until it is parallel to the pool floor and then bring the lower leg back. A companion may assist by supporting your leg under the hamstring while you flex and extend the lower leg. You may wish to sit on the edge of the pool, sit in the water on the pool stairs, or sit on a water board to perform this exercise. When sitting, both legs may be exercised at the same time. For added resistance, ankle weights or a noodle may be used. Start with eight to ten repetitions, take a few seconds to relax, and repeat the set until three sets are completed. After exercising one leg, relax a few seconds and switch to the other leg.

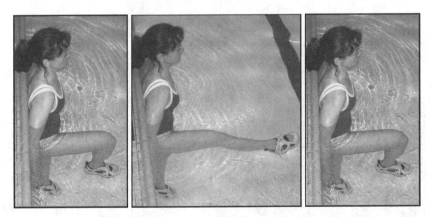

Figure 118: Quadriceps, standing

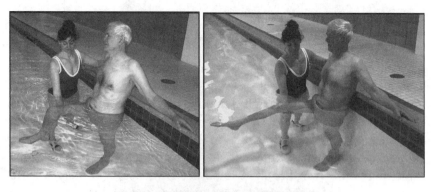

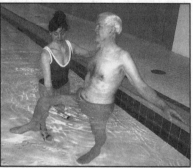

Figure 119: Quadriceps, using a partner

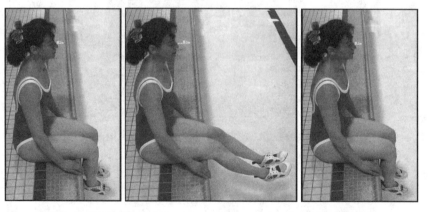

Figure 120: Quadriceps, on the pool edge, double leg

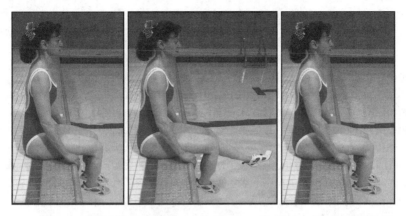

Figure 121: Quadriceps, on the pool edge, single leg

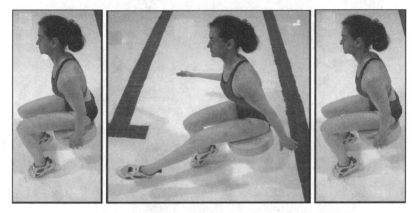

Figure 122: Quadriceps, on a kickboard

Hamstring Curl

This exercise strengthens the back of the thigh. Face the pool wall and stand in water that is waist to chest deep. Place your hands on the ledge of the pool and stand arm's length from the edge with your legs straight and feet on the pool floor. Shift your weight to the right foot and bring the left heel up toward the gluteus. Then bring the foot back to the pool floor, keeping the foot relaxed. Ankle weights may be used for added resistance. Start with eight to ten repetitions. Relax a few seconds before repeating the exercise for two more sets. After completing three sets, shift your weight to the left foot and repeat the exercise with the right leg.

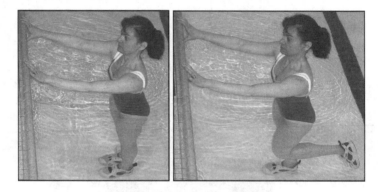

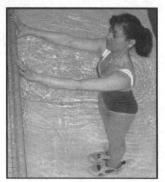

Figure 123: Hamstring Curl

Squats

Squats help to strengthen the buttocks, quadriceps, and hamstrings. Stand in waist deep water and face the pool wall an arm's length from the edge. Using the wall for balance, slowly lower yourself down as if to sit in a chair until the knee joint is as close to a right angle as possible. It is important to keep the knees right above the ankles to avoid overextending the knee joint. On the return move, contract the buttocks and the hamstrings and push the body back to an upright position. If you want to incorporate more balance into the exercise, you can balance on your feet without using the wall for support. As you assume the squat position, your arms come out in front to provide a counterbalance. One squat equals one repetition. Try to do six to ten squats per set for one to three sets.

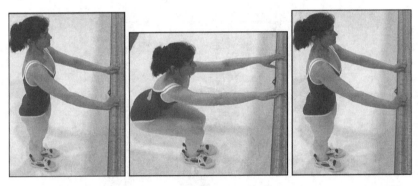

Figure 124: Squats, off the wall

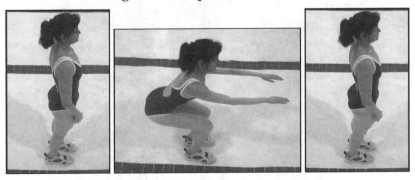

Figure 125: Squats, using the arms for balance

Lunges

Lunges help to strengthen the gluteus, quadriceps, and hamstrings but concentrate on one leg at a time. More balance is required than for Squats. Stand in waist deep water and face the pool wall an arm's length from the edge. Starting in an upright position, kneel with one leg so the upper thigh or quadriceps is perpendicular to the pool floor and the opposite leg is in a squat position. Contract the hamstrings and gluteus muscles and push through the heel of the bent leg to an upright position. Then switch to the opposite leg. The wall may be used for extra stability or you may wish to use your arms as a counterbalance in more open water. You may do six to ten repetitions on one leg before switching to the other leg or you may alternate legs until each leg has done six to ten lunges. Do one to three sets.

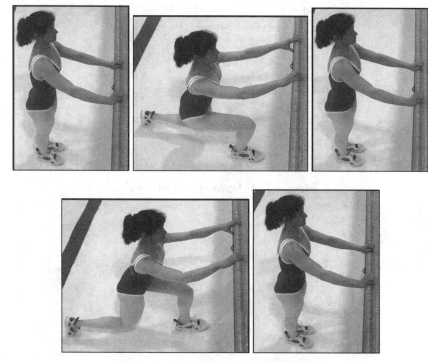

Figure 126: Lunges, using the wall

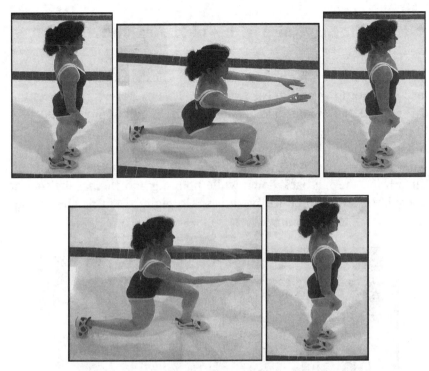

Figure 127: Lunges, using the arms for balance

Straight Leg Raise with Ankle Flexion/Extension

The calf muscle is small and the tibialis in the front of the lower leg is even smaller. It does not take much to exhaust these muscles so take care not to overdo these exercises. This exercise strengthens the calf muscle, the tibialis, and the ankle joint. Standing in waist to chest deep water with your back against the wall and using your arms for support, slowly lift a straight leg up from the hip. As you lift the leg, point and flex the foot three to five times in an alternating fashion. Then bring the leg back down while pointing and flexing the foot at the ankle another three to five times. Do eight to ten repetitions per set and work toward doing two sets in a session.

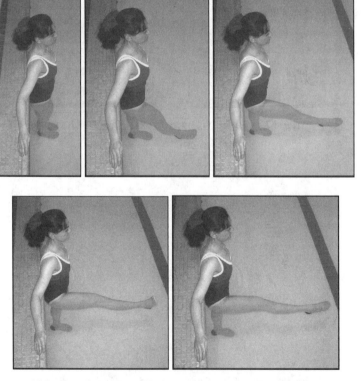

Figure 128: Straight Leg Raise with Ankle Flexion/Extension

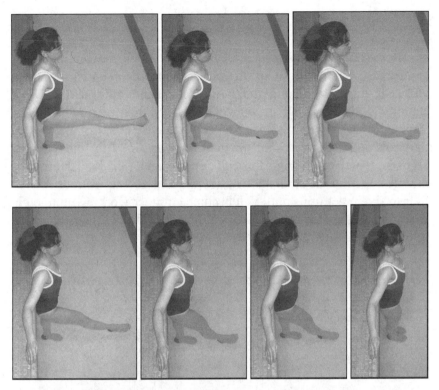

Figure 129: Straight Leg Raise with Ankle Flexion/Extension (continued)

Calf Raises

This exercise helps keep the ankle joint flexible while strengthening the calf muscle. Stand in waist to chest deep water with legs and feet together, facing the pool wall. Hold onto the wall for stability. Raise yourself up on your toes for three to four seconds. This will flex the calf muscles and extend the tibialis. Come down on the heels and lift the toes off the pool floor and hold for three to four seconds. This will extend the calf muscle and flex the tibialis, the muscle covering the shinbone. Start with just a few repetitions such as four to five repetitions until you become stronger working up to eight to ten repetitions for one or two sets. You can do both legs at a time or one leg at a time.

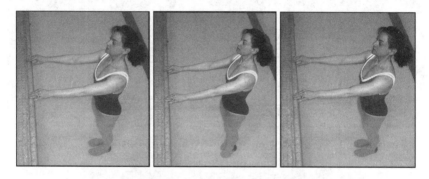

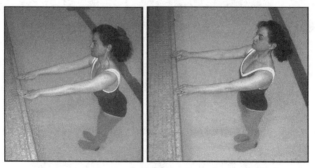

Figure 130: Calf Raise, two legs

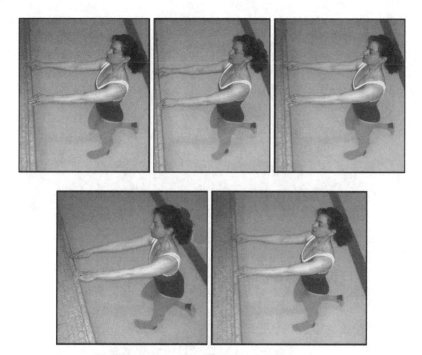

Figure 131: Calf Raise, single leg

For a more intense calf raise, you can use the pool stairs. Be sure to hold onto the pool stair railing for stability. Using the stairs will allow you to dip the heels below the level of the stairs and will bring the toes up higher flexing the tibialis more. Be careful not to over-extend the calf or over-flex the tibialis. Calf raises may be done with legs together or you may alternate the feet.

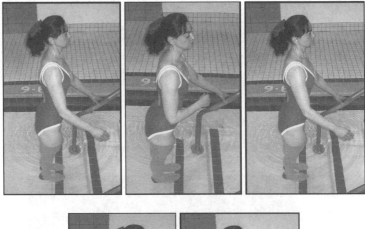

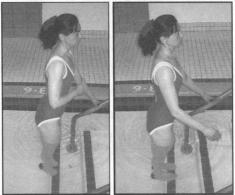

Figure 132: Calf Raises, off the stairs

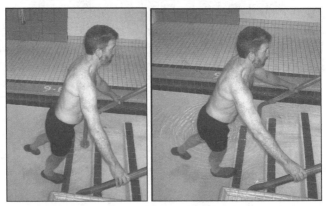

Figure 133: Single Calf Raise, off the stairs

Ankle Adduction/Abduction

This exercise helps to strengthen the ankle joint. Stand in waist to chest deep water with your back against the wall and rest your arms on the wall for support. Lift your right leg up until it is parallel to the pool floor. Flex your foot and then alternate swinging the foot toward the midline and then away from the midline for eight to ten times on each foot for one to two sets.

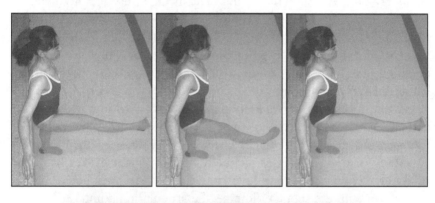

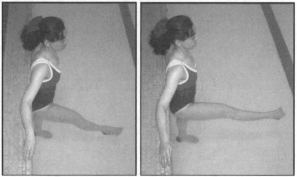

Figure 134: Ankle Adduction/Abduction

Upper Body Strength Training, Long Lever

Strength training for the upper body includes exercises for the back, chest, shoulders, arms, neck, and abdomen. The joints that are strengthened are the shoulder joints, the elbow joint, the wrist joint, and the spine. There are many daily activities that involve the neck, shoulder, elbow, and wrist joints. The neck joints are involved in activities such as reading, driving, writing, and talking. Activities involving the spine are sitting, standing, and balancing. Activities that involve the shoulder are putting on clothes, reaching for objects, combing the hair, and driving. The elbow is involved in lifting, eating, pushing and pulling items, and personal hygiene of all kinds. The wrist is used for personal hygiene, cooking, writing, and opening and closing doors and drawers. Keeping these joints supple will make living an independent life much easier.

Many of these exercises can be done with water gloves, paddles, or water weights. The long lever moves for the upper body use the whole arm with the shoulder joint as the articulation point.

Arm Cross

This exercise helps improve balance and strengthens the arms, shoulders, chest, abdominal muscles, and upper back. Stand in chest to shoulder deep water, legs straight, feet shoulder width apart, with knees slightly bent. The arms are out to the side of the body and parallel to the pool surface. To protect the lower back, you should tuck the gluteus under the pelvis. Bring your arms down from the shoulders keeping your hands cupped. Cross the arms at the wrists in front of your body at about waist height. Then lift the arms to the point of being parallel to the pool surface and bring them down from the shoulders, with hands cupped, and cross them at the wrists in back of your body, again about waist height. One crossing in front and one crossing in back equals one complete repetition. Start with one set of six to ten repetitions and then relax for a few seconds before doing another set. You should work toward three sets with ten repetitions in each set. Gloves, paddles, or weights may be used to increase resistance.

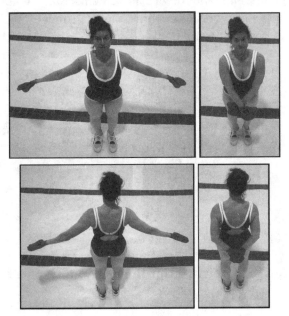

Figure 135: Arm Cross, front and back

Straight Arms Down Front

This exercise helps with balance and strengthens the arms, shoulders, abdominals, and the upper back. Stand in chest to shoulder deep water with the feet shoulder width apart, knees soft, with the gluteus tucked under the pelvis. An aquatic barbell may be used for added resistance. If you feel unbalanced, you can stand with one foot behind and off to the side. This stance provides you with a wider base of support. Hold the barbell with the hands facing down, shoulder width apart. Start with the arms and barbell just under the surface of the water. Keeping the wrists straight and pulling from the shoulder, bring the barbell down to the thighs and then, slowly and with control, bring the arms and barbell back up to just under the surface of the water. If equipment is not used, you can cup the hands. Start with the arms out in front, parallel to each other and just under the surface of the water, and turn the palms down. Then pull the arms down to the thighs, keeping them parallel to each other. Then turn the palms up and bring the arms back to just under the surface of the water. One repetition is one up and down movement. Start with six to ten repetitions in a set working toward doing ten repetitions in each set for three sets, resting briefly between each set.

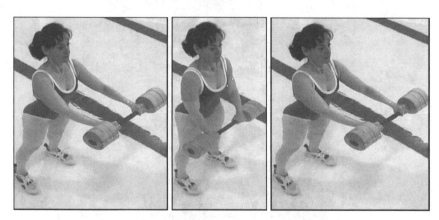

Figure 136: Straight Arms Down Front, using a barbell

An alternative way to perform this exercise is to engage one arm at a time while the other arm remains at rest in front of the body. Dumbbells or paddles may be used, one in each hand, for added resistance. The repetitions may be done in an alternating pattern of three to five repetitions with the right arm and then three to five repetitions with the left arm.

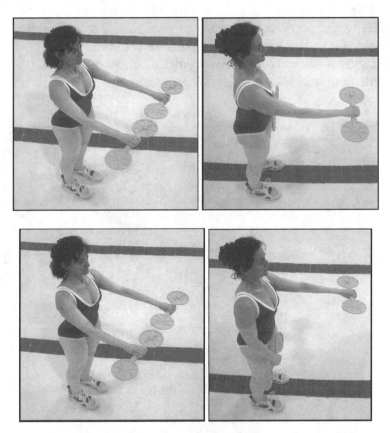

Figure 137: Straight Arms Down Front, using paddles

Straight Arm Raises to the Side

This long-lever arm exercise strengthens the back, shoulders, and chest and is done in the sagittal plane. Stand in shoulder deep water with your legs shoulder width apart and knees soft. Start the exercise with the arms at your side, hands in a cupped position and palms turned up. Slowly lift the straight arms out to the side until they are parallel to the pool surface and then reverse the palms so they are facing down and slowly bring the arms back to the starting position. Water gloves, weights, or paddles will add resistance. Do six to ten repetitions in a set. Work toward doing three sets of ten repetitions. Take brief rests between sets.

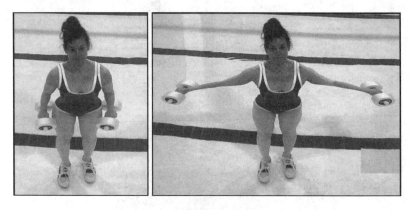

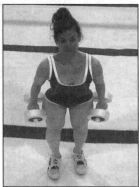

Figure 138: Straight Arm Raises to the Side

Another way for you to perform this exercise is to extend one arm at a time. You may wish to exercise the right arm for three to five repetitions and then switch to the left arm or you may wish to alternate the arms one at a time until ten repetitions are done.

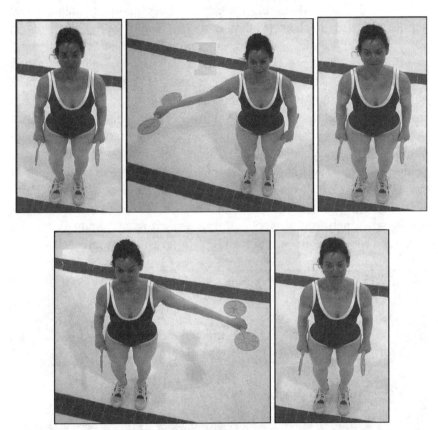

Figure 139: Straight Arm Raises to the Side, one arm at a time

Chest Flys

This exercise strengthens the muscles of the chest, abdominals, shoulders, and back and is done in the transverse plane. The muscles of the back and abdominals contract to help maintain balance and stability. Stand in chest to shoulder deep water with both arms in front, parallel to the pool floor and your hands held in a vertical position. Your feet are shoulder width apart and straight with a soft knee, or you can stand with one foot behind and to the side for a more stable base of support. If you use water weights, they should be held in a vertical position. Using the muscles of the back and posterior deltoid (the back of the shoulder), pull the arms apart and bring them straight out from your sides. Then bring the arms toward each other using the pectoralis majors (chest muscles) until they meet in front of the body again. Gloves, water weights, or paddles will add more resistance. Bringing the arms out and back is one repetition. Start with six to ten repetitions in each set and work toward doing three sets with ten repetitions in each set, taking short rests between each set.

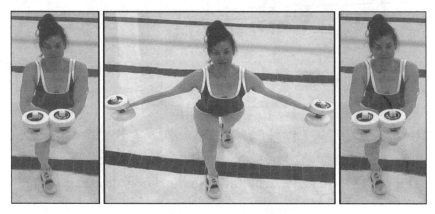

Figure 140: Chest Flys

An alternate way to perform this exercise is for you to stand with your left side to the pool wall with your left arm on the pool ledge for support and your right arm extended out in front with a soft elbow. You should have the hand held vertically or a dumbbell held in a vertical position. Move the arm in a 90° arc until the arm and hand are in line with the shoulders. Do three to five repetitions for three sets and then switches sides.

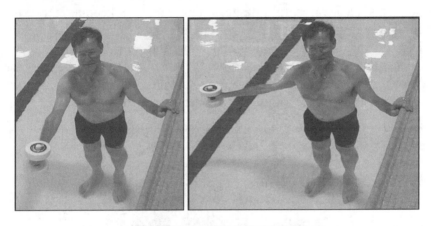

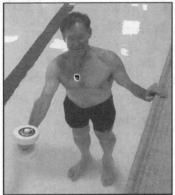

Figure 141: Chest Flys with a single arm

Arm Circles

Arm circles strengthen the shoulders and help to promote balance. Stand in shoulder deep water with feet shoulder width apart, knees soft, and the arms held straight out to the sides with the palms facing forward. For a more stable base, you can stand with one foot behind the body and off to the side. Circle the arms forward and then circle the arms backwards in a large circular motion keeping the arms straight and under control. When circling the arms, start the motion from an outstretched position and move the arms forward. As you rotate your arms, the resistance force of the water will challenge your balance. To meet this challenge, you can alter your stance, rotate the arms at a slower pace, or use the assistance of a companion.

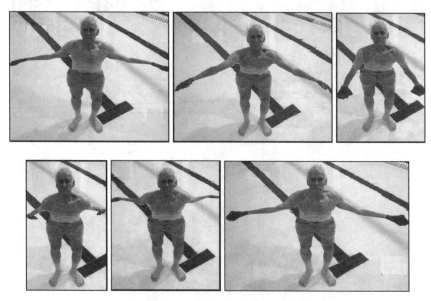

Figure 142: Arm Circles

An alternative to make it easier to keep your balance is to shorten the length of your arms by placing your hands on your shoulders before rotating the arms. Rotate the arms for a set of six to ten times forward and six to ten times backward. Rest briefly between sets and work toward doing three sets with ten repetitions each.

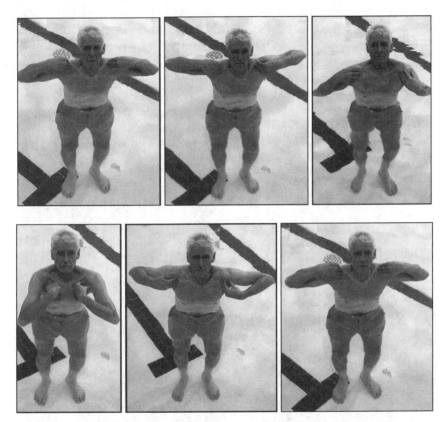

Figure 143: Arm Circles, with elbows bent

Shoulder Circles off the Pool Edge

This exercise strengthens the shoulder joint and is done from the edge of the pool. Lie prone on the outside of the pool. Leaning forward, let the arm hang down in the water. Let the weight of the arm direct the swinging just like a plumb bob, keeping the movement under control. You can also swing both arms at the same time bringing both arms toward the midline for six to ten circles and then reverse the direction working toward three sets with each arm of ten repetitions per set.

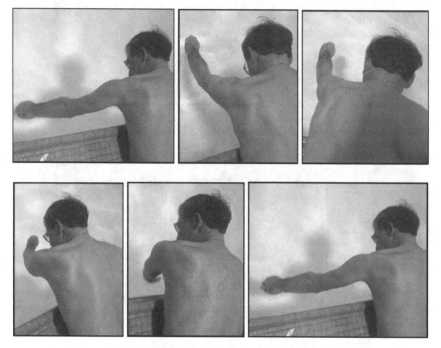

Figure 144: Shoulder Circles off the Pool Edge

Shoulder Circles in the Water

This exercise strengthens the shoulder joint. Stand in waist to chest deep water with your right hand holding the edge of the pool. Lean forward and let your left arm hang down in the water as if it were a plumb bob. Keeping the movement under control, swing the arm toward the midline for six to ten circles and then reverse the circles. After exercising the left arm, switch and exercise the right arm, working toward three sets with each arm of ten repetitions per set. Water weights are not recommended for this exercise; however, water gloves may be used.

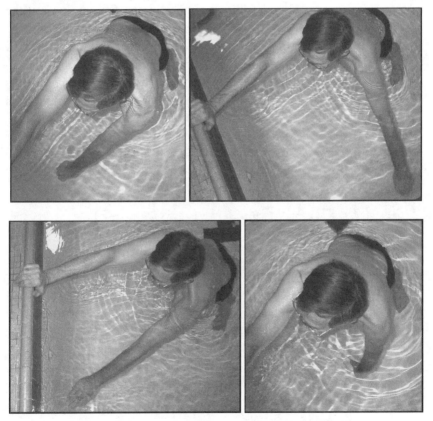

Figure 145: Shoulder Circles in the Water

Thirty-Degree Arm Raise

This arm raise exercise is done at a 30° angle and strengthens the front and back of the shoulder (the anterior and posterior deltoid). Weak shoulders promote a stooped posture, which can lead to postural instability, while strong shoulders help you maintain an upright posture and good balance. When lifting the arm up, the front of the shoulder is exercised. When the arm is returned, the back of the shoulder is exercised. As with the other arm raise exercises, stand with your feet shoulder width apart and knees slightly bent. Keep your hands open and turned at an angle with the little finger slanting upward and the thumb slanting downward so you feel a small amount of water resistance. Then lift the straight arm at a 30° angle until the arm is parallel to the pool floor and return the arm to the side of the body. When the thumb is in a downward slant, the posterior deltoid or the back of the shoulder is being exercised. If the thumb is in an upward position, the anterior deltoid or the front of the shoulder is exercised. Do six to ten repetitions working toward three sets with ten repetitions in each set and then repeat the exercise with the other arm. An alternative is to lift both arms at the same time. Since the shoulder muscles are not very big and can easily be strained, it is not advisable to use water weights.

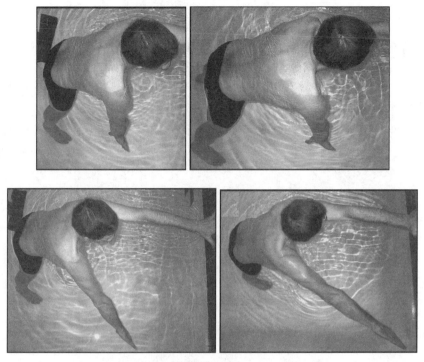

**Figure 146: Thirty-Degree Arm Raise,
single arm with the thumb down**

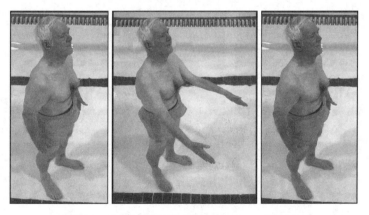

**Figure 147: Thirty Degree Arm Raise,
both arms with the thumb up**

Upper Body Strength Training, Short Lever

Short lever moves for the arms exercise the triceps, biceps, chest, shoulders, forearms, and wrist.

Wall Push-Ups

Wall push-ups help to strengthen the muscles of the biceps, triceps, shoulders, chest, and upper back and promote better posture. Stand in water that is waist to chest deep, arm's length away from the pool wall, and place your palms on the pool wall, a little more than shoulder width apart. Lean forward until the arms bend at the elbows keeping the arms parallel to the pool floor. Then push the body back from the wall until the arms are straight, being sure to keep the body in alignment from the head to the feet. The wider the arms are on the pool wall, the more the chest muscles are exercised. Do six to ten push-ups and take a few seconds to relax, working toward three set of push-ups with ten push-ups in each set.

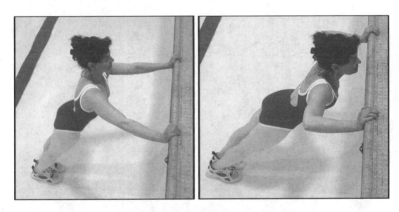

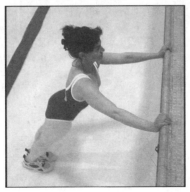

Figure 148: Wall Push-Ups

Chest Press

This exercise strengthens the shoulders and the chest. Using water weights or a larger barbell helps add resistance. Stand in chest deep water with your arms outstretched from the shoulder and bent at a 90° angle at the elbow. Your hands hold the weights or barbell in a prone position and push the weights forward until the arms are straight. Then pull the weights back until the elbows bend at a 90° angle. Each forward and backward move equals one repetition. The forearms glide a few inches beneath the water's surface and remain parallel to the pool floor. If you choose not to use weights, you will need to keep your hands flexed at the wrist and in the water in order to take advantage of the water resistance. Work toward three sets with ten repetitions in each set resting a few seconds between each set.

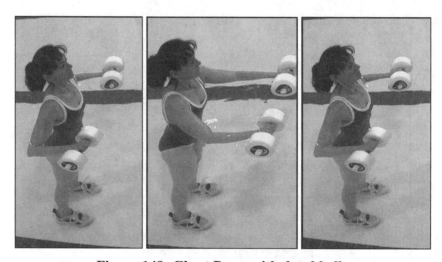

Figure 149: Chest Press with dumbbells

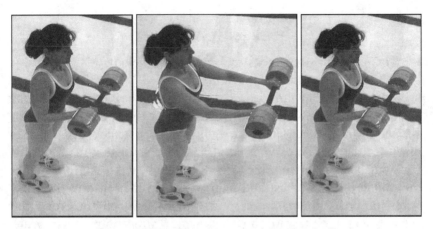

Figure 150: Chest Press with a barbell

Seesaw Arms

This exercise strengthens the shoulder and elbow joints. Stand in shoulder deep water with the arms stretched out on both sides at shoulder level with palms turned at the wrist so they are perpendicular to the pool bottom. Keep the arms at shoulder level and just under the surface of the water. Bend your right arm at the elbow and touch or reach for the middle of your chest and then straighten the right arm back out. Then bend your left arm at the elbow and reach for or touch the middle of your chest and then straighten the left arm back out. Alternate these motions for six to ten times and then relax for a few seconds and work toward three sets with ten repetitions each. Water gloves or paddles will add to the resistance.

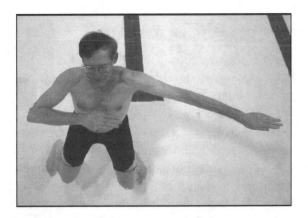

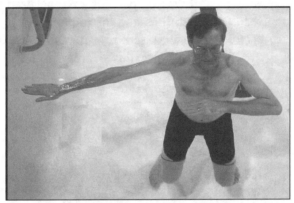

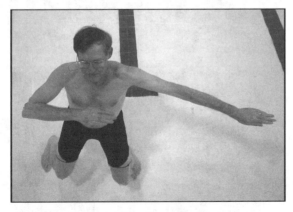

Figure 151: Seesaw Arms

Upper Arm One

This exercise works the muscles of the upper arm (the biceps and triceps). Stand in chest to shoulder deep water with legs shoulder width apart and the knees soft. Begin with your arms fully extended and by the sides of your body. The palms of the hands are turned up in a cupped position. Keep the elbows and upper arms still and close to the body as you raise the palms upward from the elbows toward the surface of the water. Turn the hands over so the palms are facing down in a cupped position and then lower the forearms until the arms are straight again. The move up works the biceps and the move down works the triceps. Water gloves or paddles may be used for added resistance. Do six to ten repetitions and then relax for a few seconds working toward three sets with ten repetitions in each set. An alternative way for you to perform this exercise is to alternate the arms, working them one at a time.

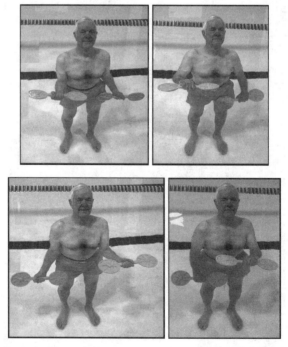

Figure 152: Upper Arm One with paddles, alternating arms

You may also do this exercise with weights, but the buoyancy of the weights results in most of the work being done by the triceps in this position. When using weights, pair this exercise with Upper Arm Two or Upper Arm Three for a balanced workout.

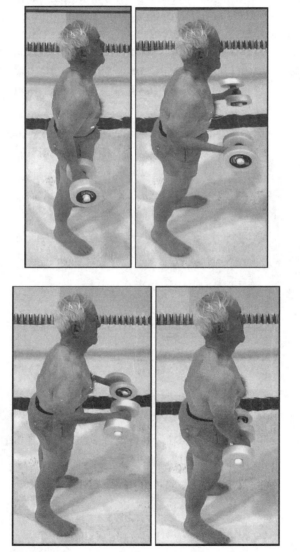

Figure 153: Upper Arm One with dumbbells, side view

Upper Arm Two

This exercise works the muscles in the upper arm. Extend your arms out to the side with the upper arms parallel to the surface of the water, bending the arms at the elbows. Pull the palms toward the center of the body. You should cup the hands and have the palms facing up when pulling the forearms in and reverse the cupped palms when pushing the forearms back out. Water gloves or paddles may be used for added resistance. If water weights are used, the biceps will be worked more than the triceps, so pair this with Upper Arm One for a balanced workout.

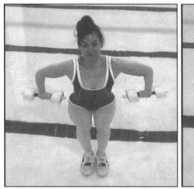
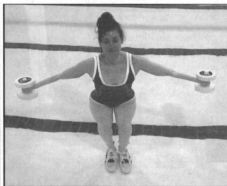
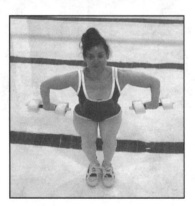

Figure 154: Upper Arm Two

Upper Arm Three

This exercise works the muscles in the upper arm. Hold the upper arms parallel to the pool floor and back behind your body. Extend the forearms from the elbows until the arms are straight, cupping the hands in a supine position when pushing back. Change the palms to a prone position when pulling the hands forward. Water gloves or paddles may be used for added resistance. If water weights are used, the biceps will be worked more than the triceps, so pair this with Upper Arm One for a balanced workout.

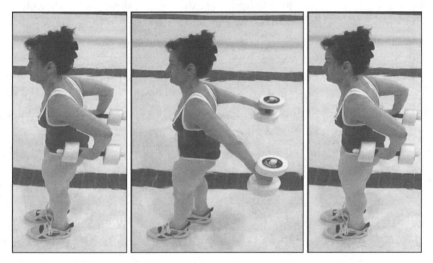

Figure 155: Upper Arm Three

Forearm Roll

This exercise works the muscles of the forearm and strengthens the elbow and wrist joint. Stand in chest deep water, with feet shoulder width apart, soft knees, the upper arm anchored to the side of the body, and the forearm extended out front with a 90° bend in the elbow. For added stability, you may wish to stand with one arm supported on the pool wall. Start with the hand in a vertical position, fingers curled in a loose fist, with the thumb pointing to the ceiling. Turn the hand at the wrist so the thumb faces the outside, and then turn the hand so the thumb faces the ceiling and then turn the hand so the thumb faces the midline of the body and then return the hand to the starting position. Do six to ten repetitions and then switch to the other hand working toward three sets on each side with ten repetitions in each set. For added resistance, water gloves or paddles may be used. If paddles are used, they should be held so they are perpendicular to the pool floor at the start of the exercise. If you feel very stable, you may exercise with both arms at the same time.

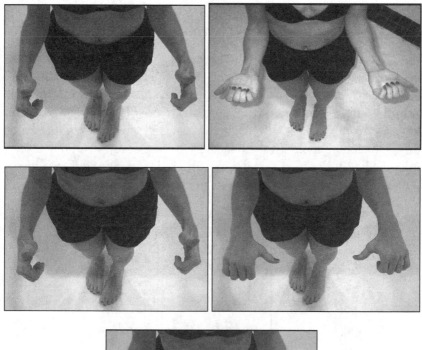

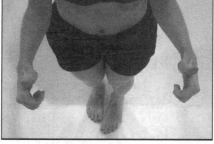

Figure 156: Forearm Roll

Wrist Strength

This exercise helps strengthen the joints of the wrist and the muscles of the forearm. Stand in waist deep water with your upper arms anchored to the sides of your body. Extend the forearms out in front from the elbows with the hands in a prone position or hold the arms down in front and just off to the side. Using water weights, water gloves, or bare hands, lift the hands up as far as they will go and then point the hands down as far as they will go. Do eight to ten repetitions in one or two sets with small breaks in between the sets.

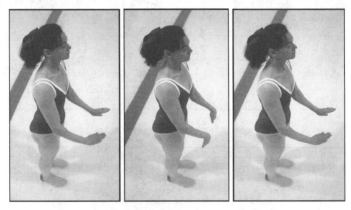

Figure 157: Wrist Strength, hands in front

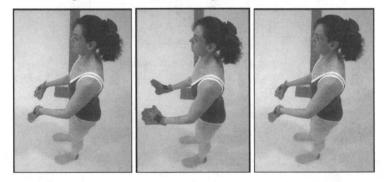

Figure 158: Wrist Strength using Water Gloves, hands in front

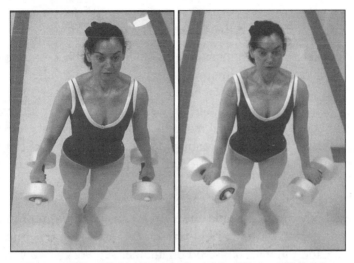

**Figure 159: Wrist Strength using Water Weights,
with hands to the side**

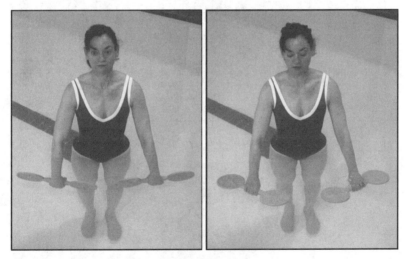

Figure 160: Wrist Strength using Paddles, with hands to the side

Elbow Arm Swing

This exercise strengthens the shoulder and back muscles and improves shoulder joint mobility. Stand in chest to shoulder deep water with your upper arm anchored to the side of your body and your forearm bent at the elbow. Hold the hand of the working arm vertical so it can act like a paddle and make the most of the water's resistance. You may wish to stand close enough to the edge of the pool to rest the other arm on the ledge for added stability. If a water weight or dumbbell is used, it should be perpendicular to the pool floor. Begin with the forearm in front of the torso and swing the forearm away from the body out to the side and then return the forearm to the front of the body. Start with the right arm and do six to ten repetitions and then relax for a few seconds and do another set working toward three sets with ten repetitions in each set.

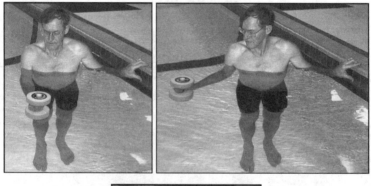

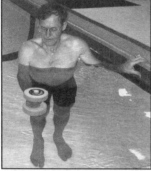

Figure 161: Elbow Arm Swing

Torso Strength Training

The torso or core muscles include the muscles of the abdomen and the back. These muscles help you move from one position to another such as moving from a reclining position to an upright position without having to use painful joints in the upper limbs. The torso muscles work in the frontal, transverse, and sagittal planes. When you are exercising the rectus abdominis (the front of the torso) and the erector spinae (the back of the torso), you are working in the frontal plane. When you are exercising the oblique muscles (the sides of the torso), you are working in the sagittal plane. Rotation exercises work in the transverse plane.

Strong abdominal muscles help keep your back straight and make it easier to walk in an upright position. Weak abdominal muscles allow the organs in the abdominal cavity to push forward, changing your center of gravity. When the internal organs protrude in front, you compensate for the added weight by swaying your back. A swayed back puts pressure on the erector spinae, causing stress and pain in your lower back. Strong abdominal muscles keep the body balanced and aligned.

Abdominal muscles do not have joints to pull against like the arm muscles and the leg muscles. To strengthen the abs, a person must contract the muscles and then work against the tightened muscles.

Rotation

This is an exercise for the oblique muscles as well as for the back muscles. Strengthening these torso muscles will help you with your balance. Stand in chest deep water with your arms extended from the shoulders, straight out in front and hands pressed together at the palms to form a paddle. Your feet are shoulder width apart with soft knees. You may keep the arms folded close to the body for less resistance. Start with the arms out in front right at the midline of the body. Without moving the hips or feet, rotate the head and the entire torso to the left using the outstretched arms and hands to capture the water's resistance. Then move the head, torso, and arms all the way to the right making a 180° arc. One arc is equal to one repetition. For added resistance, a paddle or weight may be held between the hands. Do six to ten repetitions working toward three sets with ten repetitions in each set. Take a brief rest between each set. If balance is a real issue, a partner may help you stay in a stable position.

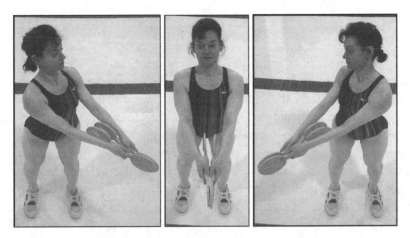

Figure 162: Rotation using paddles

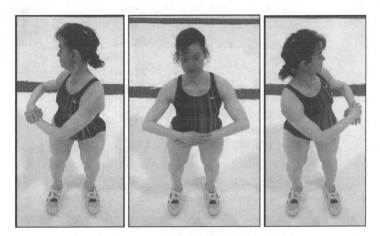

Figure 163: Rotation using folded arms

Standing Tuck

This exercise is for the stomach muscles. Stand in chest to shoulder deep water facing the pool wall and assume a neutral position with feet shoulder width apart, knees soft, chest lifted, and shoulders back. Use the pool ledge for support. Once in position, shorten the distance between the lowest rib and the hipbones by contracting the stomach muscles. This is accomplished by imagining the abdominal muscles are an accordion and the chest and the pelvis are the end parts squeezing the instrument together. Another way to visualize the exercise is to imagine the belly button being pulled until it reaches the spinal column. One contraction is equal to one repetition. Start with six to ten tucks and then work up to three sets of ten.

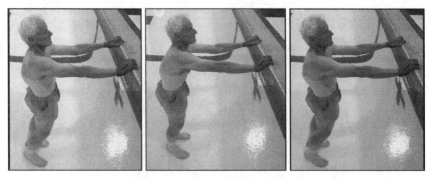

Figure 164: Standing Tuck

Supine Tuck

This is an alternative way to do an abdominal crunch. This exercise requires the use of a noodle for support. The noodle is wrapped around your upper back and held in place just under the arms. One or more noodles may be used. Lie in a supine position with your legs straight out and your head held in alignment to the neck and back. Just like the Standing Tuck, contract the stomach muscles so the distance between the lowest rib and the top of the hipbone is shortened. If your neck is stiff or sore, a partner may hold you in place and support your head. Do six to ten contractions and work toward three sets with ten repetitions in each set, relaxing a few seconds after each set.

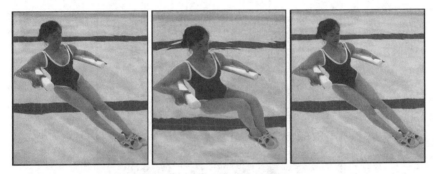

Figure 165: Supine Tuck using a noodle

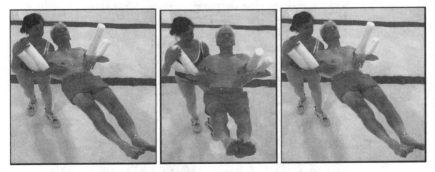

Figure 166: Supine Tuck with a partner

Side Tuck

This exercise is for the oblique muscles, which are located on the sides of the torso. Stand in shoulder to chest deep water in a neutral position with feet shoulder width apart, knees soft, chest lifted, and shoulders back. An option is to stand with your side to the wall and use it for stability. Contract the oblique muscle so that the distance between your shoulder and hip is lessened, visualizing how an accordion is squeezed. You need to be sure to concentrate on contracting the oblique muscle and not just dipping the shoulder. You can also use paddles or use the wall for support. Do six to ten side tucks on each side, working toward three sets on each side. Each set should have ten repetitions.

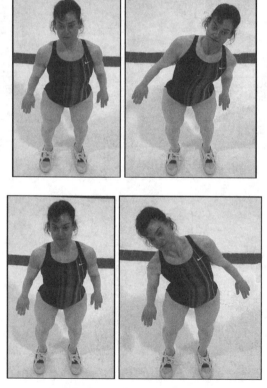

Figure 167: Side Tuck

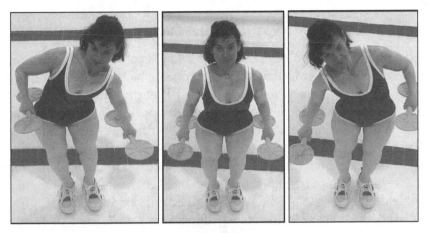

Figure 168: Side Tuck using paddles

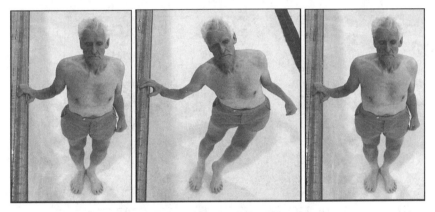

Figure 169: Side Tuck off the wall

Supine Side Tuck

This is a variation of the side tuck using a noodle for support. Lie in a supine position in the water with one or more noodles wrapped around your upper back for support. Your legs are straight out in front and your head is held in alignment with the neck and spine. Keeping your legs parallel and close together, draw the knees up toward the abs and turn them to the right. Then turn the bent legs to the midline and straighten them out. Draw your legs up again to the abs and turn the knees to the left and then bring the knees to the midline and straighten the legs. One twist to the right and one twist to the left is one repetition. Do six to ten repetitions working toward three sets with ten repetitions in each set. If your neck is stiff or sore, a partner may stand behind you and help support your head.

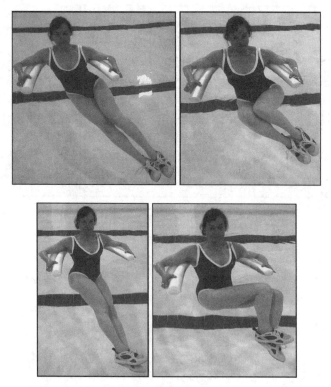

Figure 170: Supine Side Tuck using noodles

12

Cool Downs

Cool downs are a combination of flexibility exercises and stretching exercises done at a slower pace and at a less intense level. After exercising, return to flexibility exercises and do three to five repetitions. Hold and stretch the last repetition for 20 to 30 seconds so the muscle can completely relax. While stretching, do deep breathing so your heart rate returns to its resting rate. The benefits of stretching after exercising are an increased range of motion, improved joint mobility, decreased risk of muscle and joint injury, improved circulation, reduced muscle tension, improved posture, and a sense of physical accomplishment.

When cooling down, you should inhale when executing the stretch and exhale as the stretch is relaxed. During the stretch, you should not hold your breath. When stretching at the end of an exercise session, try to extend the stretch farther than when stretching at the beginning of the exercise session. If the stretch is stressful or painful, back off, relax, and try again. Since arthritis causes muscles and joints to be stiff and painful, it is not unusual for someone with arthritis to be able to stretch farther one day than another. Do not be discouraged if this should happen. Physical abilities will change on a daily basis depending on how arthritis affects you. Staying active and consistent will make you stronger and more agile in the long run.

13

Complete Plans

It is now time to put together all of the information that has been previously described into a workout plan. There are two sample plans that include warm-ups, stretching, flexibility, aerobic exercises, strength training, and cool down. The first plan for is designed to be more intense than the second plan which uses a companion. The suggested plans are designed to improve and maintain physical ability. It is hoped that these exercises will inspire a lifelong commitment to fitness as part of your overall treatment program.

With all of the examples of the individual exercises described, it is possible for fitness instructors, physical therapists, exercise partners and people with arthritis to design many more plans than those presented here. It is not necessary to include all of the exercises described in previous chapters. However, when putting together a plan, be sure to balance the body areas being trained. For example, if the plan includes strength training for the arms, it is important to include exercises that work both the biceps and the triceps. Do not exercise select parts of the body to the exclusion of others. Select a diverse and well-balance set of warm-ups and stretches so the entire body is warmed-up and ready to exercise.

People who have rheumatoid arthritis need to have strong muscles to help keep the joints aligned and the stress and pressure diminished but they also have a higher risk of cardiovascular disease so the routines are evenly divided between aerobic and strength training.

Routine #1 for Rheumatoid Arthritis

Warm-ups, 5-10 minutes
    The March
    March with Rocking Arms
    March with a Kick
    Ice Skating

Flexibility, 5-10 minutes
    Hip Circles
    Shoulder Flexibility One
    Middle Upper Back One
    Elbows
    Knees
    Wrist Circles
    Fingers
    Toes

Stretches, 5-10 minutes
    Quadriceps Stretch One
    Hamstring Stretch One
    Inner Thigh Stretch
    Calf Stretch
    Chest Stretch
    Side Stretch
    Triceps Stretch
    Finger Stretch Two

Aerobic Exercise, 15-30 minutes
    Straight Leg Aerobic Kick
    Pendulum Swing
    Cross-country Ski
    Water Run with Breast Stroke Arms
    Water Run with Rowing Arms
    Rocking Horse with Push/Pull Arms

Strength Training for Lower Body, 1-3 sets each leg with 6-10 repetitions in each set. May use water weights.
> Leg Lift Front
> Leg Lift Behind
> Side Leg Raises
> Leg Circle
> Lunges
> Quadriceps
> Hamstring Curl

Strength Training for the Upper Body, 1-3 sets with 6-10 repetitions in each set. May use water weights.
> Arm Cross
> Chest Flys
> Arm Circles
> Wall Pushups
> Upper Arm One
> Upper Arm Two, if you are using weights

Strength Training for Torso, 1-3 sets with 6-10 repetitions in each set.
> Standing Tuck
> Standing Side Tuck
> Rotation

Cool Down, 5 minutes
> The March
> March with Rocking Arms
> Shoulder Rolls
> Quadriceps Stretch One
> Hamstring Stretch One
> Calf Stretch
> Triceps Stretch
> Neck

Routine #2 for Rheumatoid Arthritis Using a Companion

Companion helps with cuing, positioning, balance, stability, and use of equipment.

Warm-ups, 5-10 minutes
Walking with Arm Swing
March
March with a Kick

Flexibility, 5-10 minutes
Shoulder Flexibility One
Shoulder Flexibility Two
Pelvic Tilt
Middle and Upper Back One
Wrist Flexion and Extension
Wrist Circles
Fingers

Stretches, 5-10 minutes
Quadriceps Stretch Two
Hamstring Stretch Two
Chest Stretch Two
Side Stretch
Triceps Stretch
Fingers One

Aerobic Exercises, 15-30 minutes
Knee Lifts
Knee Lifts with a Kick
The Water Jog
Straight Leg Scissors Cross, using the Jogging Belt
Treading Water, using the Jogging Belt

Strength Training for Lower Body, 1-3 sets each leg with 6-10 repetitions in each set. May use water weights.

Leg Circles
Leg Swing
Leg Lift Front
Leg Lift Behind
Side Leg Raises
Calf Flexion/Extension with Leg Raises
Squats
Lunges

Strength Training for the Upper Body, 1-3 sets with 6-10 repetitions in each set and on each side. May use water weights.

Straight Arm Raises to the Side
Straight Arms Down Front
Shoulder Circles off the Edge
Elbow Arm Swing
Upper Arm One
Upper Arm Three, if you are using weights
Chest Press
Chest Flys
Forearm Flexion/Extension

Strength Training for Torso, 1-3 sets, 6-10 repetitions in each set

Supine Front Tuck
Supine Side Tuck

Cool Down, 5 minutes

Low Intensity Water Walk with Swinging Arms, 30 feet
Low Intensity March, 30 feet
Shoulder Rolls, 4-6 times in each direction
Calf Stretch, hold for 20 seconds each leg
Quadriceps Stretch Two, hold for 20 seconds each leg
Hamstring Stretch Two, hold for 20 seconds each leg
Side Stretch, hold for 20 seconds each side
Triceps Stretch, hold for 20 seconds each side
Neck Rolls Side to Side, 4-6 times

An exercise log, such as this one, will help you chart your progress as well as keeping track of changes you can make to fine-tune your plan.

Exercise Log

Day	Type of Exercise	Time of Day	Medications	Results or Remarks

14

Designing a Program

While you and a companion can use the information in this book to design an exercise program, there are advantages to consulting with a professional fitness instructor or physical therapist for pre-screening and functional assessment. The professional can design a program that is tailored to your specific needs. If you and your companion want to design a program without using a professional in the field, you should at least be assessed by a physician.

Your assessment should start with a fitness evaluation checking cardiovascular functioning, flexibility, and strength. Don't be discouraged if you aren't as fit as you hoped to be. The good news is that you can improve in all of these areas by following an exercise program.

Cardiovascular Functioning: To assess cardiovascular functioning (CV), your VO2 max is measured. VO2 max is the amount of oxygen you use when performing exhausting cardiovascular work and is a good determinant of your circulatory system's ability to deliver oxygen to your body. The greater your VO2 max, the better your aerobic fitness level.

Running on a treadmill until you have reached the point of maximum fatigue is a well-known method for administering VO2 max assessment tests. Assessment of VO2 max must be done with particular sensitivity to your age and physical ability. A recumbent bike is a good tool to use if you have stiffness in your back, knees, or hips. You will be able to sit in a stable position, which reduces pressure on your back and allows you to focus on using your legs. Walking and swimming are also good assessment tools if you have trouble with balance and stiff joints.

Measuring how long it takes you to run or walk five hundred yards in the pool is another good way to assess CV. One CV test, designed at Ball State University in Indiana, uses the following steps:

Calculate the number of pool lengths (or widths) it will take to cover 500 yards. For example, in a pool that is 25 yards long you will have to cover 20 lengths of the pool.

Record how high the water is on your body so consistency in further tests can be maintained.

Record the start time and your heart rate.

Run or walk 500 yards in the water as fast as possible.

Record the finish time and your heart rate.

Take time to cool down and relax.

To determine the ideal water-depth for CV, subtract 12 to 18 inches from your height.

Improving and maintaining cardiovascular fitness should always be part of an exercise program. For the person with rheumatoid arthritis, cardiovascular fitness can be used to help decide appropriate intensity and duration of cardiovascular exercises.

Flexibility: Flexibility assessments measure your range of motion (ROM), posture, and gait. Knowing your ROM helps the fitness professional devise a program that is challenging, but not too strenuous. There are five areas that should be assessed for range of motion:

- Cervical (neck) flexion and extension
- Hip flexion and extension in the frontal plane
- Adduction and abduction in the sagittal planes
- Shoulder flexion and extension
- Elbow flexion in the frontal plane

Posture should be checked for any vertical deviations such as leaning forward or a sideways tilt. Either of these conditions could indicate stiffness in the back, hips, and knees. Exercises should be devised to help correct any problems with flexibility, balance, and posture.

The last flexibility assessment is your gait or walking posture. The assessment looks at stride length, height of the step, and how fast steps are made. Looking at the way you walk helps the person doing the assessment understand the severity of the arthritis and how it is impacting your ability to move.

Strength: Strength assessment determines the strength of the major muscle groups of the legs and arms. Knee flexion and extension and hip flexion and extension are used to assess the strength level of the legs. Shoulder flexion and extension, elbow flexion, and vertical flexion and extension assess the strength levels of the arms. Depending on your ability, one to ten repetitions should be used for this assessment. Repetition counts the number of times you can lift a certain amount of weight and what the ROM is when lifting. If you are unaccustomed to exercise, the amount of weight used may have to be as low as one pound. The fewer repetitions you can do, the less usable strength you have.

Arthritis-specific Assessments: Assessment tests specific to arthritis should also be incorporated into the general fitness assessment. Along with cardiovascular fitness, flexibility, and strength, you should also be assessed for levels of pain, inflammation, functional status, and medications.

You can assess your level of functional ability by using a scale devised by the American Rheumatism Association. This scale helps to classify people with rheumatoid arthritis by defining their level of functional ability. This scale can also be used by people with other forms of arthritis such as osteoarthritis and fibromyalgia. The scale is divided into four classifications:

Class 1:   Total functional ability. You can perform everyday activities without any handicaps.

Class 2:   Limited mobility in one or more joints, some pain but still able to perform everyday activities.

Class 3:   Functionally incapable of performing most activities.

Class 4:   Mostly incapacitated. May have to use a wheelchair or be bedridden.

A second assessment tool that is used to evaluate people with arthritis is the Arthritis Impact Measurement Scales 2 (AIMS2). The AIMS2 uses 12 different categories with scores ranging from 0 to 10,

0 representing the least impairment and 10 representing the most impairment. The categories are mobility level, walking and bending, hand and finger function, arm function, self-care, household tasks, social activity, support from family, arthritis pain, work, level of tension, and mood.

A third arthritis assessment tool is the Health Assessment Questionnaire (HAQ). It is a less extensive but still important assessment tool that measures your ability in eight categories with a range of being able to achieve the task "without difficulty" to "unable to do." The HAQ categories are dressing and grooming, rising, eating, walking, hygiene, reach, grip, and activities.

Water exercise programs should be designed to improve all areas of your life whenever possible. Emphasize increasing endurance, flexibility, and strength in ways that improve your ability to function in daily activities.

Music and Workouts

Music helps to keep you motivated as well as creating an energetic, dynamic setting for exercise. For people who are just starting an exercise program, music provides motivation as well as a distraction from the hard work. Music that has a steady, easy rhythm helps you to keep track of repetitions and sets within the exercise program. Generally, you will move to the beat of the music. The faster or stronger the beat is, the more intensely you are likely to work. Once you are moving with the music, you will become so involved with the emotional surge derived by the music and movement that the monotony of the activity will be forgotten.

At Glasgow University in Scotland, women with rheumatoid arthritis participated in a study to see if music improved exercise performance. The women who used music of their choice were able to walk 30% farther than women who did not exercise to music. The music provided just enough positive distraction so that the women exercised longer. As the popular saying goes, "Time flies when you're having fun."

In another study at Gustavus Adophus College in Minnesota, the effects of music on a person's heart rate were measured. Ten college women were asked to exercise using no music, slow music, and fast music while engaged in low, moderate, fast, and cool down exercises. The music or lack of it was introduced at random while the women exercised. The study concluded that when the music was at a faster tempo, the women's heart rates went up. This indicates that music has a definite influence on the heart rates of people as they exercise.

The type of music you use while exercising will influence your mood and will be an important factor in how pleasant and motivating your workout will be. If you like classical music, than that is what you should use. When engaged in warm-ups and stretching, music with a slow to moderate tempo is advisable. When engaged in the aerobic portion of the program, a more upbeat tempo should be used. Generally, a tempo of 124 beats per minute is used when doing the aerobics portion of the workout in the water. When doing strength training, the tempo drops to 60 to 80 beats per minute. This tempo is also good when doing the warm-ups and stretches. Music for the cool downs is generally soothing and relaxed.

Here are a few suggestions for the types of music you may wish to use. K-Tel produced a series called "Hooked on Classics" and a series call "Hooked on Swing." They also did "Hooked on Country." All have familiar musical numbers set to the background of a steady drumbeat. Michael Flately's "Lord of the Dance" has a mixture of songs that are appropriate for all phases of a workout. Other types of music would be Rock 'n Roll, Swing, Jazz, New Age, and Country Western. Whatever the music is, it has to be inspiring.

Music can be used in the format of a cassette tape or compact disc. Portable cassette tape or CD players can be set up in the pool area well away from the pool edge. It may be possible to set a player up on a stair or a chair to prevent water from splashing on the equipment. Also the acoustics may vary from pool to pool, so the sound quality may be affected. It is now possible to purchase personal headsets that are waterproof so they can be worn while in the water, but they cannot be immersed.

15

Diet

A person with arthritis needs to adopt a well balanced diet. Maintaining a nutritious, balanced diet preserves normal weight limits, eliminating excess strain and pressure on the joints. Overweight people tend to be less active, increasing their risk for chronic ailments including arthritis.

It can be challenging for a person with arthritis to achieve and maintain a balanced diet. Some people with arthritis find preparing nutritious meals difficult due to pain, limited mobility, and fatigue. Medications may cause stomach upset or diminish appetite. Pain and depression accompanying chronic illnesses can inhibit the desire to maintain good nutritional habits.

A balanced diet consists of two elements: types of foods and number of calories. The number of calories a person needs is determined by a person's age, gender, and activity level. Active women, teenage girls, and children require around 2200 calories a day. Active men, teenage boys, and very active women need around 2800 calories a day. Older adults and sedentary people need closer to 1600 calories a day. Anything less than 1600 calories a day is considered unhealthy as a maintenance diet.

The US Department of Agriculture (USDA) food pyramid shows a diet centered on consuming large amounts of carbohydrates such as fruits, vegetables, and grains; moderate amounts of meat and dairy products; and small amounts of sweets and fats. The carbohydrates are derived from potatoes, pasta, rice, bread, fruits, and vegetables. Meats include small amounts of red meat, poultry, and fish. Dairy is in the form of milk, eggs, butter, and cheese. The USDA recommended food pyramid debuted in 1992 and is quite general and simple in its approach to healthy eating. If there is a problem with the food pyramid, it is that it indicates that all carbohydrates, proteins, and fats contribute the same amount and type of nutrition to the diet when in fact they do not.

There is a reason for this. Since the 1960s the government has known of the dangers of consuming too much saturated fat and the objective of the USDA was to simplify the message about the dangers of saturated fat. They reasoned that people should replace the consumption of saturated fat with different kinds of carbohydrates.

Unfortunately, the message may have been oversimplified. In the USDA pyramid, there is no distinction made between the different types of carbohydrates. Pasta, potatoes, white bread, and white rice are not the same nutritionally as whole, unrefined grains, fruits, and vegetables. The first group contains mostly simple carbohydrates and the second group contains complex carbohydrates. In an effort to reduce ingestion of fats, food manufacturers replaced the fats found in processed foods with refined simple carbohydrates in the form of starches and sugars. This improved the taste of food since removing fats makes foods taste less desirable and it created an industry of fat-free-but–high-in-empty-calorie foods. The increased use of simple sugars and starches in processed foods has led to the explosion of obesity and type II diabetes in the last three decades. Both these conditions exacerbate arthritis.

A newer food pyramid was devised by Dr. Walter Willet of Harvard University. His pyramid differentiates between types of fats and carbohydrates and combines diet and activity.

Dr. Willet's pyramid starts with exercise at the base as the body's main maintenance source. Today people live longer and use machines to do manual work. Longevity combined with inactivity has led to a steady increase in arthritis, heart disease, obesity, diabetes, and other chronic diseases. Rather than concentrating on the next meal, scientists, nutritionists, and health care providers now believe people should concentrate on being more active. They recommend walking the dog, gardening, biking, walking, jogging, swimming, or anything that is an enjoyable activity. If you don't make exercise a regular part of your daily life, then your diet cannot benefit you nearly as much. The body will store extra calories as fat even if the calories are from nutritious food sources.

The next level in Dr. Willet's pyramid highlights whole grains and vegetable oils. Whole grain sources include oatmeal, whole-wheat bread, and brown rice. Whole grains and unrefined grain products release sugars from carbohydrates into the bloodstream at a slower and steadier rate. This fuels the body more efficiently and keeps the insulin levels steady. Whole grains and unrefined grain products are also goods sources of fiber.

Vegetable and fish oils are at the bottom of the pyramid because oils in food are a basic source of nutrition. It is important to eat the right kinds of oils that have monounsaturated or unsaturated fat. Good sources of healthy unsaturated fats include oils from olives, soy, and peanuts, as well as fatty fish such as salmon and tuna. These healthy fats actually improve cholesterol levels when eaten in place of highly processed carbohydrates or saturated fats.

The next level of the pyramid includes fruits and vegetables. There are lots of reasons to eat fruits and vegetables besides their good taste. They are a great source of vitamins, minerals, fiber, and phytochemicals. Phytochemicals are antioxidants that come from plant material. Fruits and vegetables decrease the chances of having a heart attack or stroke; protect against a variety of cancers; lower blood pressure; and guard against cataract and macular degeneration, the major cause of vision loss among people over age 65.

Nuts and legumes are the fourth layer of the pyramid. The legumes in this level include black beans, navy beans, garbanzos, and other dried beans. Nuts that are especially good for you include almonds, walnuts, pecans, peanuts, hazelnuts, and pistachios. They are all good sources of protein, fiber, vitamins, minerals, and healthy fats.

The fifth layer includes fish, poultry, and eggs. These are included as protein sources that are low in saturated fats. It may be possible to get balanced proteins from a mix of whole grains and legumes, but these protein sources are also part of a healthy diet.

The sixth layer recognizes the need to have calcium in your diet to maintain strong bones. Calcium, by itself, is not enough. You also need vitamin D, exercise, and a whole lot more. Dairy products are the traditional source of calcium in American diets, but you need to avoid as much saturated fat as you can by using low fat products. If you don't like dairy products, calcium supplements can be taken instead.

At the top of the pyramid are white rice, white bread, potatoes, pasta, sweets, red meat, butter, and other saturated fats.

The reason all of the refined grains, sugars, and potatoes are at the top of the pyramid is that the body converts white rice, white potatoes, and products made with white flour into sugar much faster than products made with wheat flour, brown rice, or whole grains. These white, refined grain products cause a rapid rise in the insulin, which the body generates to keep blood sugar levels in control. Consuming simple carbohydrates elevates the insulin level and taxes the body, especially the panaceas, making the person prone to type II diabetes, obesity, and heart disease.

An increase in insulin also suppresses the hormone glucagon. Glucagon helps the body to burn fat as a fuel. When glucagon is suppressed, protein, fat, and excess sugars are stored as body fat. Keeping insulin at an even, steady level is essential for weight control because people feel satisfied longer with the right food and will eat less.

Red meats and saturated fats should be limited because they increase low-density lipoprotein (LDL or "bad") cholesterol. For the same reason, you should avoid trans fatty acids. They are fats and oils that have been chemically altered and are found in processed foods like margarine and Crisco shortening. They are also found in prepackaged foods, donuts, cakes, cookies, and candy. You will improve your health by switching from red meat to fish or chicken several times a week. Also switch from margarine or butter to olive oil and avoid trans fatty acids.

In addition to the food pyramid, most people should take a multivitamin. It won't make up for unhealthy eating, but it can fill in the nutrition gaps that can affect even careful eaters.

Dr Willet's pyramid suggests a person maintain an active

lifestyle; consume a diet high in complex carbohydrates like fruits, vegetables, and whole grains; consume lean proteins from fish, low-fat dairy, and smaller portions of red meat. This pyramid advocates using mostly monounsaturated varieties of oils and spreads and avoiding all trans fats.

People with arthritis can and should eat a well planned, nutritious, and balanced diet; however there are certain adaptations in the diet that may help with the symptoms of arthritis.

Adaptations for Rheumatoid Arthritis:

The Arthritis Foundation recommends that people with rheumatoid arthritis consume 20-25% of their calories from protein to replace the protein lost by the inflammatory process. They should also take extra folic acid. Lean protein is an important part of the rheumatoid arthritis diet and it can be obtained by eating fish and soybean products. Folic acid counteracts the negative effects Methotrexate has on red blood cells and can be found in foods such as broccoli and in dark green leafy vegetables.

Foods that contain vitamins B, C, and E such as fruits and vegetables are beneficial for people with rheumatoid arthritis. In an Italian study reported by *Epidemiology*, vegetable consumption and the risk of chronic disease was tested. The study surveyed 46,693 people and found a strong connection between vegetable consumption and a decreased incidence of rheumatoid arthritis. A few studies indicate that people who consume diets high in vegetables and low in saturated meat have fewer symptoms of rheumatoid arthritis.

Current understanding of fats is based on studies of Mediterranean cultures. These people consume high levels of plant oils and fatty fish and yet maintain a low incidence of arthritis, heart disease, and diabetes. In a study conducted at the University of Athens Medical School in Greece, researchers found that people who consumed olive oil were less likely to get rheumatoid arthritis. Control participants were matched to people who had rheumatoid arthritis and a lifetime retrospective dietary survey was conducted on both groups. The study concluded that people who consumed the lowest amounts of olive oil had a 2½ times greater risk of developing rheumatoid arthritis than people who consumed the highest amounts of olive oil. Omega-3 fatty acids seem to have anti-inflammatory properties that inhibit the development of rheumatoid arthritis.

Flavonoids are antioxidants found in fruits, vegetables, soy products, and tea. They have anti-inflammatory effects as well as protective qualities against heart disease and cancer. Research indicates flavonoids limit inflammation associated with tissue degeneration, improve circulation, and promote collagen growth. People who consumed high amounts of fruits and vegetables, cooked or raw, had a 75% lower risk of developing rheumatoid arthritis than those who did not consume vegetables.

There are certain foods that seem to trigger rheumatoid arthritis symptoms in some people. These foods are dairy protein, corn, wheat, citrus fruits, eggs, red meat, sugar, saturated fats, salt, caffeine, and nightshade plants like potatoes and eggplant. Not all these foods will affect all rheumatoid arthritis sufferers alike. To see if these foods affect you, they need to be added or removed from your diet for three to four weeks.

For people with rheumatoid arthritis, here are anti-inflammatory dietary guidelines:
- Eat a plant-based diet.
- Eat a diet low in fats.
- Include foods that have Omega-3-fats.
- Take adequate amounts of vitamins and minerals.
- Limit sugar intake.
- Limit salt intake.
- Limit caffeine intake.
- Limit alcohol or avoid it altogether.
- Exercise regularly.
- Maintain a healthy weight.
- Keep food at a safe temperature and uncontaminated.
- Avoid overly restrictive and/or fad diets.

Research conducted in Norway and reported in a 1991 issue of *Lancet* studied the effects of diet on people with rheumatoid arthritis. Two groups of people were divided into a rheumatoid arthritis experimental group and a control group with around 25 people in each group. The study lasted a year. The experimental group ate a restricted diet that was vegetarian and excluded gluten, refined sugar, citrus fruits, alcohol, coffee, tea, salt, strong spices, and preservatives. After three to five months, low fat dairy foods were added. Researchers then added the restricted foods back into the participant's diet every second day until the end of the year. The control group ate a regular, balanced mixed food diet. Four weeks into the study, the experimental group of people with rheumatoid arthritis reported reduced swelling of the joints, less pain and pain duration, less morning stiffness, and greater grip strength. These changes lasted throughout the study. This study suggests that a vegetarian diet with the proper amount of protein made positive changes in the symptoms of rheumatoid arthritis. Two years later 45 of the original group were reexamined. Those who remained on the dairy-vegetarian diet maintained their improvement.

Some people with rheumatoid arthritis have difficulty cooking and eating because of pain in the joints of their hands. People will cook and eat what is easy to handle even if it is not as nutritious as other types of foods. It is easier to eat prepared foods that are prepackaged rather than cut, peel, chop, and assemble a plate of vegetables when you have hands that are painful and uncooperative. The problem is most prepackaged foods are not as nutritious as raw or fresh foods. Poor nutrition can lead to weight gain, putting stress on the joints. Exercise and proper nutrition are important for flexible and agile hands.

Water

One of the most important parts of any diet is water. The general rule among fitness professionals and nutritionists is a healthy person should drink a least eight 8-oz. glasses of water a day. It is believed that drinking coffee, tea, or soda does not count as liquid intake because these drinks act as a diuretic and cause a person to excrete too much liquid.

This belief stems from an interpretation of a report conducted in

1945 by the Food and Nutrition Board that found a healthy body requires 1 ml. of water for each calorie consumed. That equates to eight 8-oz. cups of water for 2000 calories. The report also stated that most of the necessary liquid is contained in existing foods. For example, tomatoes are 94% water, milk is 90% water, and even a meal of dry bread and cheese contains 35% water. The notion that a person must consume eight additional glasses of water a day beyond what is obtained through other means comes from remembering and repeating "eight glasses of water for every 2000 calories consumed." The rest of the study has unfortunately been forgotten.

To illustrate the point that all liquids are equal in relieving dehydration, a study was conducted at the Center for Human Nutrition in Omaha, Nebraska. Researchers gave 18 healthy men in their 20s and 30s eight glasses of water or eight glasses of equal amounts of soda, coffee, tea, and water and recorded their hydration levels. The study showed that no matter what combination of liquids the men drank, their hydration level was the same. Water is still the best choice for hydration because water is calorie free, but other beverages do not diminish the benefits of hydration. The only beverage that can be considered a "negative" beverage is alcohol because the liver requires one 8-oz. glass of water to process one ounce of alcohol.

Water helps the body to metabolize fats and can reduce the risk of bladder infections and bladder cancer. The more water the kidneys and liver receive, the easier it is for those organs to break down and excrete non-essential fats. A lack of enough water causes the liver to store fats rather than to break down and process fatty acids. Hydration helps prevent urinary tract infections because bacteria are not able to attach to the bladder lining. It also helps reduce the risk of bladder cancer. The *New England Journal of Medicine* reported the risk of bladder cancer was reduced 7% for every 8 oz. of water consumed.

In another study reported by the Fred Hutchinson Cancer Research Center in Seattle, women who drank four 8-oz. glasses of water a day cut their risk of colon cancer in half as compared to women who consumed only two 8-oz. glasses per day. The researchers concluded that increased amounts of water enable waste products to move faster through the gastrointestinal tract reducing the amount of time waste remains in the bowel and reducing the chance for problems to develop.

Too much water can also be a problem. If you drink more water than your kidneys can handle, you may suffer water intoxication. This occurs when electrolytes in the body become so diluted that physical changes, behavioral changes, or even brain damage can occur. According to urologists, the best way to know if you are getting enough water is to check the color of your urine. As long as you are in good health and the urine is clear to pale yellow, you are getting enough water.

16

Alternative Remedies

Although conventional medicine, which involves a relationship between you and your doctor, is the mainstay of the western world, alternative medicine also has something to offer. Alternative medicine believes your mental and physical environment play an important role in your health.

Alternatives that Work

There are seven basic alternative remedies that are recommended for people with arthritis.

1. Self-help courses. These are educational courses offered by the Arthritis Foundation and others. They provide information on coping skills, support groups, and general information about arthritis. When you know more about your disease and the treatments available, you feel more empowered and less frustrated with your situation. Medicine is not the only way to improve your health. These courses will help you find good alternatives.

2. Mind/body therapies. These are techniques used to relieve pain, depression, stress, and anxiety. You learn deep breathing and relaxation techniques that help improve your overall condition. Getting in touch with your body helps you understand how what you do makes a difference in how you feel.

3. Yoga, Tai Chi, and Qigong. These practices help improve balance, mood, and strength by exercising the mind and body at the same time. The exercises involved can be specifically tailored to help relieve arthritis symptoms and promote overall better health. Many people find these forms of exercise more enjoyable than standard Western exercise programs. Choose the form of exercise you can stick with.
4. Acupuncture and acupressure massage. Acupuncture originated in ancient China. Hair-fine needles are inserted into specific points on the body with pressure or with mild electrical pulses. Acupressure uses the same points in a more massage-like setting. Acupuncture and acupressure are used to treat pain and relieve muscle tightness.
5. Massage. Massage is a passive treatment used to help sooth sore muscles and release tension. It is particularly helpful if your muscles are too sore to exercise or if you are stuck in a pain-tension-pain cycle. When the muscles are relaxed through massage or other manipulations like aquatic therapy, joints can move with much less pain, leading to better sleep, which, in itself, can be healing.
6. Dietary supplements. Rheumatologists urge caution when considering supplements. The supplements rheumatologists recommend most are glucosamine, chondroitin, and Omega-3 oils found in fish and flaxseed. These supplements help your body deal with the pain, stiffness, and cartilage deterioration caused by arthritis.
7. Exercise. Of all of the alternative therapies, exercise (Eastern or Western) has proven to be the most beneficial. Appropriate exercise makes you feel better, look better, and physically perform better. As long as you avoid exercise during flare-ups and don't seriously overdo it, there should be no negative side effects. Exercise is also the hardest therapy for people to maintain because it takes dedication and determination. Find the kind of exercise that works best for you.

Any alternative remedies should be discussed with your doctor before you try them. Many people with arthritis are nervous about approaching their doctors about alternative therapies. Responsible physicians are informed about alternative medicine and stay current with new information so they can provide the best care. Here are some suggestions you can use when talking with your physician about alternative therapies:

- Be positive. Don't assume the doctor will have a negative reaction about other therapies. Most doctors are receptive to your concerns and welcome your willingness to make an effort to get better.

- Allow sufficient time. Doctor's visits can be brief, so schedule enough time for a thorough discussion.

- Come prepared. Research the therapy or therapies before talking with the doctor and, if possible, bring information for the doctor to evaluate.

- Listen to your doctor. If your doctor approves of using an alternative method, that's great. However it is also very important to listen if the reaction is negative. Your doctor has your best interests in mind. Do not tune doctors out just because they may not approve of a therapy that sounds promising. Ask why they disapprove of the therapy. It may be the method is harmful, dangerous, or illegal. It is the doctor's job to know about available therapies and their effects.

- Keep records. If an alternative therapy is used, keep accurate records of the effects of the treatment. Make sure these records become part of your conventional medical record. This is especially important if you are using fish oil or herbs that can interact with other medications. Accurate records keep traditional and nontraditional methods from counteracting each other.

- Don't keep secrets. Always tell your doctor if you are taking other medications or using other treatments besides what the doctor has prescribed. This should include all over the counter medications, vitamins, diets, or exercise. Doctor/patient relationships are based on trust and respect. If you are not truthful with your doctor, then the best care isn't possible.

- It is possible your doctor won't agree with a treatment you think would be effective, so it may be necessary to find another doctor who is more open-minded. It is not wise to totally abandon conventional medicine, but you should be able to find a doctor who is more willing to blend approaches.

Unproven Remedies

As long as there has been arthritis, there have been those who claim to have a cure. There are a lot that don't work and some that are even deadly. Let's take a look at a few of them. Then there will be some suggestions about how to evaluate claims, which will help you decide whether you want to investigate a treatment further.

In 1796, Elisha Perkins invented one of the earliest gadgets claiming to cure arthritis. He called it the "Perkins tractor." Perkins claimed that a surplus charge of electricity in the body's fluids caused a number of conditions especially gout, pleurisy, violent insanity, yellow fever, inflammatory tumors (arthritis), and rheumatism. The Perkins tractor consisted of two pointed rods three inches long. One was gold colored and the other was silver. By drawing the tractors over the affected areas, Perkins claimed electricity supposedly trapped in the body's fluids would be released.

For some reason, practitioners of dubious remedies often link electricity to the cause of arthritis. In the 20th century, there have been a number of electrical devices confiscated by the FDA. In 1954, the Palorator was a gadget with two electromagnetic coils that vibrated a couple of knobs on a box sending out a so-called healing current. Other such contraptions are the Gonsertron and the Magnetron. Both use electrical currents to vibrate chairs. Vibrating gadgets are another favorite gimmick that unscrupulous people use to entice people to try their products. The danger is that vibrating chairs and mattresses do nothing for arthritis and keep people from seeking effective treatment. In the meantime, the disease progresses and gets worse.

The use of unproven remedies by people with arthritis is a big business costing people with arthritis and their families over a billion dollars per year. According to the National Council against Health Fraud, 95% of people with arthritis will use some form of self-treatment even after they have seen a physician. Symptoms of arthritis have periodic remissions. During remissions, pain and swelling can disappear for days, weeks, months, or even years at a time. These remissions convince people their arthritis is cured and whatever treatment they were using was responsible for the cure.

Unproven remedies are treatments that lack scientific backing or medical viability. In order for a remedy to be proven, unbiased, scientific tests are needed to validate the authenticity of the product or practice. Some treatments are considered health frauds when there is no scientific data to support the claims and often, there is scientific data that refutes the claims. Some treatments may be beneficial but are so new there has not been enough time to test them thoroughly. These treatments may be on the market even though they are still being studied. The responsible course of action with these particular remedies is to acknowledge the unproven status and advise caution until more study has been done. Unknown remedies that are not being studied or tested should send up a red flag to anyone considering their use.

Treatments for arthritis must prove their validity by passing scientific tests. They should avoid stress and damage to joints and meet one or more of the following requirements:
1. Keep joints moving safely
2. Reduce pain
3. Reduce inflammation
4. Maintain or improve a person's ability to function independently

Arthritis treatments and products must also address these three questions:
1. Which type of arthritis is this remedy for?
2. How safe is the remedy?
3. How is the remedy promoted?

If a remedy claims to work on all types of arthritis, other health problems, cites only one study, cites a study without a control group, or uses testimonial histories rather than unbiased scientific evaluations, then it should be questioned.

Since there are many types of arthritis that are quite different from one another and since people with different types of arthritis use very specific medicines, it is not logical that one remedy would work for many different types of arthritis and also other unrelated aliments such as diabetes and cancer. A remedy that is truly safe and effective will be cited in more than one study and will be measured against a control group in order to eliminate any doubt of its value. These studies should be easy to locate and replicate.

Remedies relying only on testimonials cannot be tested or studied by independent parties and should be suspect. Testimonials are often characterized by claims with only a first name or just initials at the end of statements. Since the names are incomplete, the truth of the testimony cannot be verified. If people are pictured, there is no way to verify if they are who they claim to be.

The safety of a remedy is suspect if there are key pieces of information missing about the product or practice. That information would be:

- A lack of instructions, warnings, or possible side effects listed on the container
- Claims to be safe, and/or claims to be natural with no other supporting information
- No list of ingredients

When remedies are advertised, they should list relevant information such as what type of aliment the remedy helps, what is in it, how to use it, how long the effects last, and what, if any, side effects to expect. Suspicious remedies are those that claim to cure arthritis, claim to be based on a secret formula, are only available from one source, or can only be purchased by mail order or through the media.

Many people do not seek treatment or receive improper treatment for arthritis because they are confused and overwhelmed by the abundance of information available, or they hold onto deeply held unfounded beliefs. Among these beliefs are

1. Nothing can be done about arthritis
2. There are severe side effects from legitimate drugs and medications
3. There is a cure-all

Let's confront these misconceptions one by one.

1. Nothing can be done. There are many options for treating the symptoms of arthritis. The most important treatment step is seeing

a physician and being properly diagnosed so that the most effective treatment can be started and supervised by a qualified specialist. Some of these treatments include prescription medication, surgery, diet and exercise or a combination of these. These options successfully treat the symptoms of arthritis but they do not cure arthritis. Treating the symptoms effectively makes living with arthritis easier.

2. Severe side effects. Although alternative therapies are being used more and more, they are not necessarily safer or better than conventional therapies. The terms "herbal," "organic," or "natural" are not synonymous with "safe," "effective," or "free of side effects." The FDA does not regulate herbal and dietary substances and the manufactures of these products are not required to prove their treatments work or that they are safe. The Dietary Supplement Health and Education Act (DSHEA) is a law passed by Congress in 1994. DSHEA weakened the control of the FDA and allows herbs produced as dietary supplements to be considered safe unless proven otherwise. DSHEA has allowed the herbs-as-medicine market to grow. Herbs, supplements, and their claims are not subjected to clinical trials and tests like pharmaceuticals. Manufacturers of herbal medicines are not required to disclose or record complaints by consumers. Therefore, if adverse reactions occur, there is little legal recourse for the public. There are side effects from conventional medicines and there are side effects from alternative medicines. Conventional medicines, in general, are more thoroughly tested. Some have been used effectively for hundreds of years.

3. The cure-all. Most people with arthritis understand they have a treatable but incurable condition. People with arthritis must learn to live with their condition and find the treatment or combination of treatments that provides the most relief. The search for such treatments can be tedious, frustrating, and even discouraging. Many people with arthritis self-medicate to save on the cost of medicines and visits to the doctor. This can lead you to seek unproven measures in order to find satisfaction.

The best treatment for arthritis requires an accurate diagnosis by a physician as to which of the over 170 types of arthritis you have. Once the diagnosis is established, a treatment program can be tailored to fit your needs. This is very important since the disease, treatments, and remedies vary from person to person.

Until a cure for arthritis is found there are legitimate, proven remedies and treatments that offer temporary or even long-term relief from the symptoms. A claim of a cure is not only irresponsible, but fraudulent. There are no secret formulas, no cure-alls. Scientist and researchers share their knowledge about arthritis with each other so that new treatments can be reviewed and processed safely and quickly. Anyone claiming to have a secret formula or claiming to be the sole provider is misleading you. Doctors, nurses, scientist, and researchers and their families are afflicted with arthritis just like the rest of the population. They are sincerely interested in the best remedies for themselves, their families, friends, and patients.

17

Frequently Asked Questions

This chapter includes questions about several types of arthritis and fibromyalgia. Many people also have fibromyalgia or more than one type of arthritis, so I decided to include a wider range of the questions I am asked.

I have osteoarthritis. Can I pass this on to my children?

Genetics seem to be a contributing factor in 30% of people who have osteoarthritis in their hands and 65% of people who have osteoarthritis in their knees. Researchers have found a higher incidence of osteoarthritis between parents and children and among siblings than between people who are not genetically related. Other researchers have found that the breakdown of cartilage is sometimes promoted by a genetic defect. This damage allows harmful enzymes to penetrate the collagen and accelerate the destruction of the cartilage. The abnormal structure of the collagen meshwork seems to allow excess water to accumulate as well, which can cause painful swelling and pressure. A study was reported in a 1998 issue of *Arthritis and Rheumatism*, where 337 families were studied to see if osteoarthritis is inherited through a major recessive gene that is passed to children from either parent. Of the sample, 51% of the parents had osteoarthritis and 33% of their offspring had osteoarthritis in one of the joints of the hand. Dr. Bjorn Olsen, a cell biologist at Harvard University, has been studying the genetic possibilities of osteoarthritis for 10 years. Olsen has been able to identify three genetic variations in people with osteoarthritis that make the cartilage more vulnerable to degeneration when excess pressure is applied.

Is rheumatoid arthritis an inherited condition?

A person is three to five times more likely to develop rheumatoid arthritis if either of a person's parents or a sibling has rheumatoid arthritis, but no one knows why.

Is fibromyalgia inherited?

The cause of fibromyalgia is generally unknown; however, physical or emotional trauma may be implicated in the development of the syndrome. As mentioned earlier in the book, some people may have abnormal pain transmission responses. It has also been suggested that sleep disturbances may cause the condition. There are other theories that suggest fibromyalgia is caused by a decrease in blood flow causing weakness and chronic fatigue. Pilot studies have shown a possible inherited tendency toward developing fibromyalgia especially among first-degree blood relatives, but the evidence is very preliminary.

I have osteoarthritis of the knee, and walking is difficult, will water exercises help?

When you are in the water, you are more buoyant and your joints are relieved of weight and pressure that can cause pain. Once you are free of the discomforts of the compression in your joints, exercise becomes easier. It is important for people with osteoarthritis of the knee to strengthen the quadriceps so they can walk and remain independent. Having weak quadriceps, the muscles in the front of the thigh, increases the risk of osteoarthritis of the knee. Dr. Kenneth Brandt, a rheumatologist at Indiana University, studied a group of 400 elderly people and discovered that having weak thigh muscles preceded the onset of osteoarthritis. Stronger muscles take the pressure off of the joints limiting the amount of damage done to the cartilage. A strong quadriceps also maintains the space between the bones more effectively. In a normal X-ray of a joint, a wide space between the bones can be seen. In advanced osteoarthritis, the joint space is diminished due to cartilage loss and the bone is rough and condensed. Although people with osteoarthritis need to strengthen and maintain strong quadriceps, they should do so only if their knees are in good alignment. Dr. Leena Sharma of Northwestern University found that people with misaligned knees or unusually loose knees had to be extra careful when engaging in strength exercises for the quadriceps. For people with these conditions, maintaining strength in the upper thigh should be the objective. Many of the walking and quadriceps exercises presented in this book will help to strengthen the quadriceps as well as to promote balance and cardiovascular endurance.

Does smoking increase a person's risk of getting arthritis?
Smoking seems to be a significant environmental factor for people who develop rheumatoid arthritis. According to Dr. Charles G. Helmick, smoking every day increases a person's risk of arthritis by 60%. More specifically, smoking among women makes them more susceptible to rheumatoid arthritis. Another related smoking factor that is affecting how much a person is at risk for arthritis is directly related to the amount of GSTM1 that is in a person's body. GSTM1 is an enzyme that helps to detoxify cancer-causing agents often found in the environment. Many such agents are present in tobacco. Among Africans and African-Americans, 75% to 80% of the population is born with a high level of GSTM1. Only 45% to 50% of Asian and Caucasian populations are born with GSTM1. A lack of GSTM1 or a low level of GSTM1 is directly related to an increased risk of getting rheumatoid arthritis.

Another reason smoking may determine the severity of rheumatoid arthritis is because smoking has a negative affect on the immune system. The body of a person with rheumatoid arthritis produces autoantibodies that attack the body's own antibodies, particularly the IgG antibody. Autoantibodies are also called "rheumatoid factor." Sixty to eighty percent of people with rheumatoid arthritis test positive for rheumatoid factor. The chemicals found in tobacco are thought to damage the antibody IgG prompting the body to produce more rheumatoid factor. When the gene GSTM1 is present, this does not seem to be the case.

People with rheumatoid arthritis, who lacked the gene GSTM1

and who were smokers or previous smokers, were more likely to have rheumatoid factor. The number of years a person smoked was also proportional to the amount of rheumatoid factor in their system. Those who did not smoke but lacked GSTM1 were less likely to test positive for rheumatoid factor. The study showed that among the women with rheumatoid arthritis, the joint damage was just as severe among those who had quit smoking after being diagnosed, as those who continued to smoke.

Is chronic myofascial pain related to fibromyalgia?

The pain associated with fibromyalgia is often referred to as chronic myofascial (CMF) pain. The relationship of fibromyalgia and CMF is reciprocal because the symptoms of one ailment amplify the symptoms of the other and the two perpetuate each other making treatment difficult.

Belonging to a fitness center or community center is expensive. So is a trainer or therapist.

The average cost of an individual fitness membership is $60 to $80 per month. Exercise provides a way to defer, reduce, or eliminate the cost of long-term care. Joining a fitness center or community center provides an environment that promotes physical activity and it can also serve as a social outlet. Remaining physically and socially active are key elements in remaining independent and happy.

Long-term care is also costly. More than half of the U.S. population will require long-term care in their lifetime. The average cost of living in a nursing home is $50,000 per year. The average cost of in home visits from a nurse is $100 a day or roughly $3000 a month. The fitness center may be a bargain.

I have rheumatoid arthritis and was wondering if water exercise will help to relieve the tired feeling that I get throughout the day.

Water exercise helps the brain release endorphins that produce a euphoric, energized feeling. The water also helps to cushion the joints making exercise more enjoyable. At the Jean Mayer USDA Human Nutritional Research Center on Aging at Tufts, Dr. Ronenn Roubenoff compared 23 people with rheumatoid arthritis to 23 people without rheumatoid arthritis. He found that the people with rheumatoid arthritis had accelerated metabolisms and less body cell mass (the part of the muscle that is not water). People with rheumatoid arthritis have changes in their metabolism that cause their bodies to consume their own muscle. Dr. Roubenoff found that if people with rheumatoid arthritis did strength training, they could counter the loss of muscle by increasing the muscle mass and by reducing the self-consuming actions of their metabolism. They also had improved function and overall feelings of well-being.

Will arthritis medications interfere with maintaining a balanced diet?

Yes. There are certain medications that affect how well the body uses food. Glucocorticoids, which are used in the treatment of rheumatoid arthritis, can cause a person to lose potassium and to retain sodium. People with both rheumatoid arthritis and osteoarthritis often take antacids to reduce stomach irritation. These antacids may also contain high levels of sodium, calcium, and magnesium. If a person has kidney problems, it will be harder for the body to regulate these minerals. It is important for you to consult with your physician about your medications and diet and whether it is necessary to include or avoid particular supplements.

Can a person get arthritis from other environmental causes?

Yes. One example is the association between exposure to mineral oil and the risk of developing rheumatoid arthritis. This was found in a study done in Sweden from 1993 to 2003. A population-based study of cases of people with rheumatoid arthritis found that among the men exposure to mineral oil as part of their work was associated with a 30% increase in the risk of developing rheumatoid arthritis.

I have rheumatoid arthritis and am trying to eat a balanced diet but I am confused by many of the food labels. Some food products claim to be natural but still have unusual ingredients listed. Why?

Foods labeled "natural" may still contain artificial preservatives, coloring, flavoring, and other additives. One trick that manufactures use is to claim that a product such as American cheese is a natural product. The cheese is natural but the rest of the product may legally contain artificial substances. Here is a brief breakdown of some of the more common labels:

Sugar free: These are products that contain no sugar but may contain sweeteners such as corn syrup, fructose, dextrose, or honey, which are all simple carbohydrates and contain calories.

Reduced calorie: This means the food product must contain 1/3 fewer calories than a comparable product. If blue cheese dressing contains 300 calories per serving, then reduced calorie blue cheese dressing would have 200 calories per serving.

Low calorie: A low calorie product cannot have more than 40 calories per serving. Check the serving size to see if it is realistic.

No preservative: This means exactly what it says. There are no preservatives, but artificial colors and flavors are allowed.

Fortified and enriched: Often when food is processed some of the nutrients that were present in the beginning are lost and have been replaced. However, not all of the lost nutrients are replaced in the refined product. This is especially true of breads and flour.

Most foods are required to list their ingredients on a label. The ingredients are listed in order according to their weight in the final product. If sugar is listed first then it is the main ingredient.

Is it possible to have osteoarthritis and rheumatoid arthritis at the same time?

Yes. Joints damaged by rheumatoid arthritis are more susceptible to osteoarthritis.

What is the difference between osteoarthritis and osteoporosis?

Osteoporosis and osteoarthritis are both diseases that are characterized by bone density problems. Osteoporosis is characterized by the loss of bone mass which leads to low bone density and osteoarthritis is characterized by increased bone density and bony growths called osteophytes along with the degeneration of cartilage. Both conditions can be disabling and water exercises can help. For people with osteoporosis, the resistance and drag properties of the water help rebuild the weakened bones. These same properties of water also help strengthen the muscles and tendons that surround the joints affected by osteoarthritis.

Why should I exercise?

Arthritis is one of the most common reasons people have for becoming inactive. Arthritis is a painful condition and, when people are in pain, it is hard to be inspired to exercise. However, people who are active, including people who have arthritis, are healthier and live longer, more enjoyable lives than people who are inactive. People with arthritis who are sedentary are less fit, weaker, and less flexible. As a result they suffer more pain due to the complications of inactivity such as muscle atrophy, obesity, poor sleep, and the vicious cycle of pain and fatigue that accompanies it.

Once a person has arthritis, how long does it last?

Most types of arthritis are chronic, therefore arthritis and the treatments for it last a lifetime. People with some types of immunogical arthritis such as rheumatoid arthritis often have periods of remission when the symptoms of the disease improve or disappear. Remissions may last a long time, but not forever.

Is arthritis fatal?

Arthritis in itself is not fatal, but people who have arthritis, such as rheumatoid arthritis, can have an increased risk of other diseases. People with rheumatoid arthritis are at an increased risk for cardiovascular disease. This is because they have higher levels of homocysteine than other people. High levels can irritate blood vessels leading to blockage of the arteries or atherosclerosis. High homocysteine levels also cause the creation of low-density lipoprotein or LDL cholesterol. High levels of homocysteine are caused by a lack of adequate amounts of vitamin B12, B6, and folic acid.

A report at the annual congress of the European League Against Rheumatism (EULAR) in 2001 showed that people with rheumatoid arthritis were 70% more likely to die of heart disease and 30% to 40% more likely to suffer acute blockage of the blood vessels as compared to people with osteoarthritis. People with rheumatoid arthritis were 60% more likely to suffer from a thromboembolic event as compared to people without arthritis. There are theories that link arthritis and heart disease but the cause for the increase in heart disease among people with rheumatoid arthritis is still not fully understood. One thought is that inflammation which is central to the effects of rheumatoid arthritis somehow has a major role in the blockage of blood vessels and in atherosclerosis, the progressive narrowing and hardening of the arteries.

How can I get started on a water exercise program?

You need to discuss exercise options with your doctor. Once your doctor has diagnosed which arthritis you have, he or she may want you to start off with a physical therapist or fitness trainer. Check with the local health clubs, community centers, or the YMCA/YWCA for water fitness programs that are tailored to people with arthritis.

What water temperature is best for a person with arthritis?

The water should be between 83°F and 90°F.

Where can I find an arthritis support group?

Contact the local office of the Arthritis Foundation. The toll free number is 1-800-568-4045. You can also use the Internet and find message boards and bulletin boards to make contact with other people.

Are there organizations where I can get more information about arthritis and fibromyalgia?

Yes, there are many fine organizations devoted to arthritis and fibromyalgia education and treatment.

Arthritis Foundation
1330 West Peachtree Street
Atlanta, GA 30309
1-800-568-4045
www.arthritis.org

The American College of Rheumatology
1800 Century Place, Suite 250
Atlanta, GA 30345-4300

404-633-3777
www.rheumatology.org

National Institute of Arthritis and Musculoskeletal and Skin Diseases
(NIAMS)
Information Clearinghouse, National Institutes of Health
1 AMS Circle
Bethesda, MD 20892
877-22NIAMS (226-4267)
www.nih.gov/niams/healthinfo

International Association for the Study of Pain (IASP)
909 NE 43rd St., Suite 306
Seattle, WA 98105-6020
206-547-6409
http://www.iasp-pain.org

For people with rheumatoid arthritis:
American Autoimmune Related Diseases Association Inc.
22100 Gratiot Ave.
East Detroit, MI 48021
586-776-3900
www.aarda.org

18

Conclusion

At some point in our lives, most of us will have to deal with the onset of some form of arthritis. Water exercises can help lessen the limitations caused by this disease. Numerous studies have shown that people who have rheumatoid arthritis gain enormous benefits from engaging in water exercise programs. The water helps to cushion the joints that are affected by rheumatoid arthritis and helps you maintain balance and coordination. Keeping fit helps you maintain the ability to sense your body's position, reducing the incidence of falling and incurring injuries.

Water exercises incorporate the properties of drag, resistance, viscosity, and hydrostatic pressure, which help you to strengthen your muscles without placing stress or strain on your joints. Keeping joints flexible and retaining a full range of motion will help you maintain an independent life style for a long time.

Glossary

abdominals the group of muscles on the front of the torso, below the chest and above the pelvis. Also called rectus abdominis.

abductors muscles that are used to lift a body part away from the midline of the body. The hip abductors are on the outer thigh.

acetaminophen a non-analgesic drug and one of the nonsteroidal anti-inflammatory drugs (NSAID) used in the treatment of osteoarthritis. It is available over the counter and without a prescription. (See NSAID.)

acupuncture Chinese technique using needles to pierce certain areas of the body to relieve pain.

adductors muscles that are used to pull a body part toward the midline of the body. The hip adductors are on the inner thigh.

aerobic with air or oxygen.

aerobic exercise activities that can be done without depleting the oxygen in the muscles. When the body is engaged in aerobic exercise, energy is being produced with oxygen from the bloodstream. The cardiovascular system is being used at around 60% to 80% of its maximum capacity, but it can replenish the oxygen while the exercise is going on. Good for burning fat and strengthening the heart and lungs.

anaerobic exercise activities performed at a high enough intensity that the body can't supply sufficient amounts of replacement oxygen while the exercise is taking place.

analgesic a drug that reduces the body's response to pain and/or relieves pain.

angiogenesis the formation of new blood vessels.

ankylo- prefix meaning bent or crooked; used to refer to stiffening of the joints.

ankylosing spondylitis a particular type of arthritis, which first affects the spine.

antibody protein produced by the body's lymphocytes to fight foreign proteins called antigens. (See antigen.)

antigen a foreign carbohydrate complex or protein that causes an immune response from the body.

antigen-presenting cell a white blood cell that finds a foreign or invading organism, digests it, and presents an antigen on its cell surface.

antioxidants substances such as vitamins A, C, and E and minerals such as zinc, copper, and magnesium. Believed to destroy the free radicals that scientists think are responsible for mutating the body's cells thus causing cancer, cataracts, and the aging process.

antipyretic fever-reducing.

arachidonic acid unsaturated, fatty acid found in animal fats or synthesized in the body from a dietary source of linoleic acid. One of the eicosanoids.

Arava disease-modifying antirheumatic drug that inhibits the formation of the immune cells that cause inflammation.

arthralgia pain in a joint.

arthritis one of approximately 200 rheumatic diseases characterized by chronic joint inflammation, stiffness, swelling, and redness. May affect one or more joints.

arthrocentesis procedure that removes synovial fluid from a joint.

arthrography x-ray procedure that shows a detailed image of a joint by injecting air or a contrasting substance into the joint space.

arthron Latin prefix meaning joint.

arthropathy joint disease or joint disorder.

arthroplasty surgical procedure to restore integrity and function of a joint.

arthroscopy procedure where a small incision is made so a camera can be inserted into the body to aid in the examination of the interior of a joint.

articular cartilage tissue covering bone surfaces in moving joints.

autoimmune disease condition characterized by inflammation and tissue destruction caused by the body's immune system reacting against its own organs and tissues.

ball and socket joint the most mobile type of joint in the body allowing the arms and legs to move in all directions with articulation points in the shoulder and hip.

biceps muscle located along the front of the upper arm; used to bend the arm at the elbow.

B lymphocyte white blood cell which produces antibodies.

BMI Body Mass Index.

body fat the part of the body that is comprised of fat cells.

Bouchard's nodes bony spurs that occur in the middle joints of the fingers.

buoyancy upward force that a fluid exerts on an object that is less dense.

bursa protective, fluid-filled sac between bones and ligaments, tendons, and muscles.

bursitis inflammation of the bursas resulting in swelling and pain.

calorie a unit of heat that is equal to the amount of heat needed to raise the temperature of one kilogram of water one degree Celsius at room temperature; usually used as a measure of the amount of energy in foods.

carbohydrates group of organic compounds that include sugar, starches, gums, and cellulose that serve as the body's major fuel source in an average American diet.

cardiovascular system for moving blood that involves the heart and blood vessels.

cartilage resilient connective tissue which covers and cushions the ends of the bones in a joint and absorbs shock.

cartilaginous joint also called sliding or gliding joint; a tough cartilage plate joining two bones that allows slight movement; found in the vertebral column.

Celebrex one of class of non-steroidal anti-inflammatory drugs called COX-2 inhibitors; no longer available.

chondrocyte cell that forms cartilage in the body.

chondroitin amino acid used in connective tissue. Supplements containing chondroitin are used to treat arthritis.

collagen main structural protein in connective tissues.

collagenase enzyme that breaks down collagen.

complex carbohydrates carbohydrate with a complex chainlike structure that takes the body longer to turn into simple sugars. Examples are fruits, vegetables, and whole grains. Complex carbohydrates offer a more sustained level of energy over simple carbohydrates.

connective tissue material that holds the various body structures together. Blood vessels, cartilage, tendons, and ligaments are made up of connective tissue.

cool-down slowing down at the end of an exercise program to allow the body's temperature and heart rate to gradually decrease.

corticosteroid potent anti-inflammatory hormone made naturally in the body or synthetically for use as a drug. Used to treat osteoarthritis.

COX short for cyclooxygenase.

COX-1 enzyme natural enzyme made by the body that protects the lining of the stomach.

COX-2 enzyme natural enzyme made by the body that causes arthritis inflammation.

COX-2 inhibitors class of non-steroidal anti-inflammatory drugs used to block the COX-2 enzyme.

crepitus crackling sound or grating sensation in a joint; may be caused by swelling or bone surfaces rubbing against one another.

cyclooxygenase (COX) enzyme that oxidizes arachidonic acid to prostaglandin.

cytokine "messenger" molecule that enables cells to communicate and change one another's function.

dehydration depletion of body fluids; detected by dark, concentrated urine, persistent thirst, and dry mouth.

deltoids group of three muscles wrapped around the top of the shoulders; used to lift the arms forward, backward, and to the side. Also used to rotate the arms inward and outward.

diagnosis determination of the nature of an illness through patient interview, physical examination, and laboratory testing.

disease-modifying anti-rheumatic drugs (DMARD) class of drugs used to slow the progression of rheumatoid arthritis.

edema condition where the body retains fluid.

eicosanoids group of substances that are derived from the arachidonic acids.

elastin stretchable protein found in connective tissue.

ellipsoidal joint found at the base of the fingers; allows flexion/extension and limited side to side movement.

endorphins chemicals found in the brain that are released during exercise and contribute to an uplifting feeling often referred to as the "runner's high."

enthesis place where ligaments attach to the bones.

enzyme protein that speeds the rate or regulates the chemical changes or reactions in other substances.

erythrocyte sedimentation rate (ESR) diagnostic test used to indicate the presence of inflammation by measuring the rate at which red blood cells settle to the bottom of a test tube. When swelling and inflammation are present, the blood proteins bunch together and become heavy. The faster these proteins fall to the bottom of a test tube, the more severe the inflammation.

fibromyalgia chronic condition that includes widespread pain in the muscles and soft tissues surrounding the joints, accompanied by fatigue.

fibrous joint also called a fixed joint; found in joints that don't allow movement such as the bones of the skull.

flare-up reoccurrence or worsening of symptoms.

flavonoids molecular compounds found in many foods that come from plants.

flexibility range of motion around a joint. Flexibility can be increased with careful, consistent stretching and range of motion exercises.

gastrointestinal (GI) referring to the stomach and intestines.

gene small basic unit containing the codes for inheritance. Genes occupy specific places on the chromosomes.

genetic referring to one or more genes.

genetics study of heredity.

gliding joint compound hinge joint allowing movement up and down and side to side; found in the ankle and wrist.

glucagon fat-burning hormone. Glucagon is produced by the pancreas in response to adequate amounts of protein in the diet.

glucosamine amino acid used in connective tissue. Supplements containing glucosamine are used to treat arthritis.

glucose a simple sugar.

gluteus maximus, medius, and minimus three muscles of the buttocks and hips. Used to extend the thighs forward and to the side and used to rotate the legs at the hips.

glycogen the form carbohydrates take when stored in the muscles.

gout form of arthritis caused by urate crystals deposited around the joints.

hamstrings group of muscles located on the back of the thighs between the hips and the knees; used to bend the leg at the knee.

Heberden's node bony growth found on the joint closest to the fingertip.

hereditary referring the passing of genetic traits from parent to child by means of the genes.

hinge joint connection between bones that allows movement back and forth like a swinging door; found in the elbow, knees, toes, and fingers.

homocysteine amino acid produced in the body. In high levels homocysteine leads to blockage in the arteries. People who have rheumatoid arthritis usually have higher levels than people without rheumatoid arthritis.

human leukocyte antigen (HLA) type of receptor on cells that are involved in the recognition of foreign antigens. Some of the antigens are associated with arthritis.

hyaluronic acid lubricating substance found in normal joint fluid.

hydrogenate infusing hydrogen into an unsaturated fat in order to make liquid fat solid.

hydrostatic pressure pressure from water that is exerted on the surface of an immersed body.

immune system combination of organs, cells, and naturally produced chemicals that protect the body from foreign substances, diseases, and infection by identifying the abnormal cells or invaders and attacking them.

immunosuppressant reducing the effectiveness of the immune system; the name of a class of drugs used to treat rheumatoid arthritis by inhibiting the anti-immune character of the disease.

infectious arthritis arthritis caused by invading microorganisms that infect the joint fluid and tissues.

inflammation redness; immune system's protective response to tissue damage.

injury damage to the body. Symptoms include redness, pain, swelling, and heat.

insulin hormone secreted by the pancreas that helps the body to metabolize carbohydrates and regulate blood glucose levels.

irritable bowel syndrome (IBS) recurrent periods of abdominal pain, diarrhea, and/or constipation.

isometrics form of exercise where opposing muscles are contracted and held to increase the tone of the muscle fibers.

-itis Latin suffix meaning inflammation.

joint place where two bones meet.

keratoconjunctivitis sicca (dry eye) persistent dryness of the eye which sometimes occurs in people with rheumatoid arthritis.

lactic acid byproduct of high-intensity or anaerobic exercise. Lactic acid collects in the muscles and causes soreness.

latissimus dorsi pair of muscles that extend across the middle and lower back and attach the arms to the spine; used to pull the arms down and back.

lefunomide one of the Arava drugs. See Arava.

leukotriene chemical involved in inflammation and blood flow.

lift chair method of pool entry using a chair or sling that swings into position over the pool and lowers a person into the water.

ligament tough, elastic tissue that connects two or more bones and keeps them in alignment.

lymphocyte type of white blood cell.

lymphoproliferative disorders variety of disorders involving the lymph system.

macrophage type of phagocyte or white blood cell found in the bloodstream and tissues which removes bacteria, foreign invaders, and damaged tissue from the blood or tissues.

methotrexate anti-cancer drug that is effective in lower doses as a slow-acting anti-rheumatic drug.

misoprostol synthetic prostaglandin used to prevent gastric ulceration in people who take nonsteroidal anti-inflammatory drugs.

moveable floor method of pool entry using a floor that raises or lowers thus lifting a person from or submerging a person in the pool.

neutrophil white blood cell that fights infections; a phagocyte.

nodule solid "lump" or node in soft tissue.

NO-NSAID nitric-oxide releasing non-steroidal anti-inflammatory drug. Used in the treatment of rheumatoid arthritis.

Non-Steroidal Anti-Inflammatory Drug (NSAID) class of drugs that reduce prostaglandin by inhibiting cyclooxygenase. NSAIDs reduce the symptoms of arthritis such as pain, redness, inflammation, and swelling. Examples are aspirin and ibuprofen.

NSRISs norepinephrine serotonin reuptake inhibitors; used in the treatment of fibromyalgia.

obesity excessive body weight due to an accumulation of fat.

obliques muscles that are located along the sides of the torso. The external obliques are located from the lower ribs to the pelvis and allow forward bending and twisting at the waist. The internal obliques are located from the hips to the lower ribs and lie underneath the external obliques. The internal obliques allow the body to bend and rotate at the waist.

ossification process of bone production.

osteoarthritis most common form of arthritis characterized by the loss of joint cartilage, joint space, and formation of bone spurs. Commonly occurs in the knees and hips. Symptoms include pain, stiffness, and loss of movement in the joint.

osteoarthritis of the hip type of osteoarthritis most common in men, usually appearing between the ages of 20 and 60.

osteoarthritis of the knee form of osteoarthritis most common in middle age women; associated with obesity.

osteophyte outgrowth of bone.

osteoporosis progressive deterioration of bone density.

pannus proliferation of synovial tissue.

pectorals pair of muscles in the chest used to pull the arms toward or across the chest.

perceived exertion level of intensity a person feels when exercising. On a scale of 0 to 10, a perceived exertion of 6 to 7 is within aerobic limits.

phagocyte white blood cell that engulfs and ingests bacteria and other foreign molecules allowing waste cells and materials to be removed from the body.

pivot joint joint that allows turning movement such as side to side, nodding, or up and down; found at the base of the skull.

placebo inactive substance used in controlled studies to help determine the effectiveness of a tested product.

platelet disc-shaped blood particle that causes blood clotting.

prone lying face down

proprioception body's awareness of place or position of joints produced by internal sensations.

prostaglandins class of lipids present in tissues and bodily fluids that contribute to the proper function of the stomach and intestinal lining, platelets, and kidneys. Prostaglandins are also responsible for inflammation and inhibition of gastric acid secretion.

quadriceps group of muscles located on the front of the thigh. Used to straighten the leg at the knee.

ramp method of pool entry. Ramps can be permanent or removable. They allow for a gradual sloping entry along the side of a pool.

Raynaud's phenomenon condition where blood vessels constrict and cause fingers and toes to become sensitive to cold temperatures. Often seen in people with fibromyalgia.

reactive arthritis joint problems caused by viral or bacterial infection elsewhere in the body.

remission period in which symptoms of a disease diminish or disappear.

repetition single movement, as in doing one arm curl.

resistance force water's ability to exert force against movement in all directions.

rheumatic disease any of the 170 disorders that cause chronic joint pain, inflammation, or deterioration of the joints, muscles, or bones.

rheumatic factor antibody found in the blood of about 80% of people with rheumatoid arthritis.

rheumatism pain and stiffness of soft tissues in the joints.

rheumatoid arthritis crippling form of arthritis; an autoimmune disorder that is characterized by chronic pain and stiffness in the joints.

rheumatoid factor protein found in the blood of most people with rheumatoid arthritis.

rheumatologist doctor who specializes in the treatment of arthritis.

rheumatology branch of medicine devoted to the study, research, and treatment of arthritis.

rhomboids muscles connecting the base of the neck to the inside edges of the shoulder blades; used to pull the shoulder blades inward.

rofecoxib (Vioxx) one of the class of drugs of non-steroidal anti-inflammatory drugs called COX-2 inhibitors; no longer available.

SAARDs slow-acting anti-rheumatic drugs. Similar to DMARDs; used in the treatment of rheumatoid arthritis.

sacrum large triangular bone at the base of the spine.

salicylate drug made from salicylic acid that reduces inflammation, pain, and fever. Aspirin is the commonly used form of salicylate.

serotonin neurotransmitter that helps people fall asleep.

set number of repetitions of a movement, such as an arm curl. For example, a set may have six repetitions.

simple carbohydrates carbohydrate that consist of only one or two units that are easy for the body to break down. Simple carbohydrates supply the body with quick energy that does not last long. Examples are sugar, honey, refined starches, and candy.

Slow-Acting Anti-Rheumatic Drug (SAARD) class of drugs that slow or stop the progression of rheumatic disease. An example is methotrexate.

spurs bony growths that project outward from the ends of a bone in a joint. A common condition found in people with osteoarthritis.

SSRI class of drugs used in the treatment of fibromyalgia.

static stretch simple stretch that is held steadily for several seconds without moving.

substance P neurotransmitter that helps in the transmission of pain impulses along the nervous system.

supine lying on the back, face up

susceptibility having a greater than normal vulnerability to a disease.

symptom indications of a disease that can be seen or measured by others.

synovial fluid translucent, sticky fluid that acts as a lubricant in freely moving joints. It is secreted by the synovial membrane and found within the joints and bursa.

synovial joint most mobile type of joint. Examples are the shoulders, wrists, fingers, and hips.

synovial membrane (also called synovium) the lining of a joint capsule. The membrane releases a fluid that allows the joint to move more easily.

synovitis inflammation of the synovium.

target heart rate level of intensity in which the heart is being exercised but not overworked. A good target heart rate is 60% to 85% of a person's maximum heart rate.

T lymphocyte white blood cell that interacts with B lymphocytes and destroys abnormal cells.

tender points sensitive areas for people with fibromyalgia, found in specific locations on the body. Also called trigger points.

tendon strong, fibrous band of tissue that connects muscle to bone.

tendonitis inflammation of a tendon, usually caused by injury. It restricts the movement of the muscles that are attached to the tendon.

transfer stairs method of pool entry using moveable stairs connected to a platform that allows a person to transfer from a wheelchair to the pool by sliding down the stairs.

trapezius muscles that stretch from just below the back of the head, down the upper spine to the shoulder blades and collarbone. Used along with the deltoids to lift the arms and shoulders.

triceps muscles along the back of the upper arm; used to straighten the arm at the elbow and to push the arm forward.

trigger points see tender points.

type II diabetes acquired form of diabetes precipitated by obesity, stress, menopause, and other factors.

tryptophan amino acid found in milk, meat, and fish that raises serotonin levels in the brain.

ulcer non-healing break in the mucous membrane of an organ.

vasculitis inflammation of the blood vessels.

Vioxx non-steroidal anti-inflammatory drug; COX-2 inhibitor; no longer available.

VO2 max The largest volume of oxygen the body can take in and use. "V" is for volume and "O2" is for oxygen. The more fit a person is, the higher the VO2 max will be.

warm-up gentle, slow exercises done at the beginning of an exercise session to prepare the muscles, heart, and lungs for activity.

weight-bearing exercise exercises where a person supports his/her weight or lifts weight. Such exercises help to offset bone loss and osteoporosis.

x-ray electromagnetic energy used to produce images of bones and internal organs onto film.

zero-depth entry method of pool entry where the pool floor starts at the same level as the pool ledge and gradually slopes down to a deeper level.

Bibliography

Anderson, D. (1996). *50 ways to cope with arthritis*. Lindwood: Publications International.

Arthritis diet and importance of dietary supplements. (2005). (Online), February 18, 2005 from http://www.living-with-osteoarthritis.com/html/diet.php3

Arthritis Foundation (Producer/Director). (1992). *PEP-Pool Exercise Program*. [Video Tape]. Pleasant Hill, CA: Arthritis Foundation.

Bailey, C. (1999). *The ultimate fit or fat*. New York: Houghton Mifflin Company.

Baker, L. (2000, November). Fish oil, vitamin E help arthritis symptoms. *University at Buffalo Reporter, 32,* 1.

Baker, S. (2002, January/February). Does coffee, tea or soda count? *Arthritis Today, 16,* 19-20.

Bartlett, S. (2002). (Online) Management, osteoarthritis and body weight. September 4, 2003 from John Hopkins Arthritis at http://www.hopkins-arthritis.som.jhmi.edu/mngmnt/osteoandweight.html

Bauer, J. (2001, October). Can diet therapy relieve fibromyalgia? *RN, 64,* 22.

Bennett, R., Clark, S., Campbell, M., & Burckhardt, C. (1992, October). Low levels of somatomedin C in patients with the fibromyalgia syndrome: A possible link between sleep and muscle pain. *Arthritis and Rheumatism, 35,* 1113-1116.

Berne, K. (2002). *Chronic fatigue syndrome, fibromyalgia and other invisible illnesses*. Alameda, CA: Hunter House Inc.

Bjerke, M. (1997). *Examination of disability and impairment based on the ICIDH criteria in a fibromyalgia population: The impact of aquatic exercise*. Dissertation. College of St. Catherine, St. Paul, MN.

Brackett, M. (1999). *The effect of aquatic exercise on symptomatic pain felt by fibromyalgia patients.* Thesis. University of Maine, Farmington, MA.

Brainum, J. (1992, June). Mega hurts: Fibromyalgia means living in constant pain but exercise may help. *Muscle and Fitness, 53,* 167-180.

Brewer, E. & Angel, K. (2000). *The arthritis sourcebook.* Los Angeles: Lowell House.

Carling, D. (1995). *The effect of water activity on the flexibility and perceived self-efficacy of rheumatoid arthritis patients.* Dissertation. Utah State University, Logan, UT.

Cartmell, J. (2001, November). Fibromyalgia: A plausible model for cause and cure. *Townsend Letter for Doctors and Patients, 220,* 38-40.

Christ, P. (2001, Summer). Drink to good health. *Ostomy Quarterly, 38,* 38.

Clegg D., Reda D., Harris C., et al. (2006). Glucosamine, Chondroitin Sulfate, and the Two in Combination for Painful Knee Osteoarthritis. *New England Journal of Medicine, 354*:795-808.

Cline, J. (1989). *Effect of land and water exercise on hip and knee flexibility in female osteoarthritis elderly. (Exercises, hip flexibility).* Dissertation. California State University, Long Beach, CA.

Colby, K. & Kendrick K. (1987). *The effects of the Arthritis Aquatic Program on arthritic adults.* Dissertation. San Jose State University, San Jose, CA.

Copeland, B. & Franks, B. (1991). Effects of types of intensities of background music on treadmill endurance. *Journal of Sports Medicine and Physical Fitness, 15,* 21-23.

Cox, B. (Producer). (1993). *Aqua exercise for arthritis, arthritis series 1* [Video tape]. Santa Maria: Rothhammer International Inc.

Cypress Bioscience, Inc. announces Topline final results of Milnacipran phase II study in fibromyalgia syndrome. (2003, February, 10). *Business Wire,* 0216.

Daniels, D. (2000). *Exercises for osteoporosis.* New York: Hatherleigh Press.

Danneskoild, S., Lyngberg, K., Risum, T., & Telling, M. (1987). The effect of water exercise therapy given to patients with rheumatoid arthritis. *Scandinavian Journal of Rehabilitation Medicine, 19,* 31-35.

Darrow, T. (1990, January/February). Make a splash! The benefits of water exercise. *Arthritis Today, 4,* 16-20.

Dellapena, D. (2002, January). Tune out painful joints: Make exercise easier despite arthritis pain. *Prevention, 54,* 63.

Duncan, K. (2002). Vegetarian diets in the treatment of rheumatoid arthritis.

(Online), March 12, 2003 from Vegetarian Nutrition at www.andrews.edu/NUFS/arthritis.html

Dunkin, M. (2001, June). The benefits of water exercise. *Arthritis Today, 15,* 27.

Dunkin, M. (2001, June). Your medicine. *Arthritis Today, 15,* 36-39.

Dunkin, M. (2002, January). Arthritis Today's 2002 drug guide. *Arthritis Today, 16,* 32-51.

Ellert, G. (1985). *The arthritis exercise book.* Chicago: Contemporary Books.

Essert, M. (n.d.). Why water works. (Online). September 9, 2002 from Aquatic Therapy, Aquatic Rehabilitation, Aquatic Resources Network at http://www.aquaticnet.com/fibromyalgia.htm

Eustice, C. (2004). Joint hypermobility and fibromyalgia. (Online), September 9, 2004 from http://www.arthritis.about.com/cs/jh/a/hypermobfms.htm

Exercise Prescription for Fibromyalgia. (2001, October). *Prevention, 53,* 78.

Felson, D., Ahang, Y., Anthony, J., Naimark, A., & Anderson, J. (1992, July). Weight loss reduces the risk for symptomatic knee osteoarthritis in women: The Framingham Study. *Annals of Internal Medicine, 116,* 535-540.

Feltham, K. (1994). *The effects of a 6-week water exercise program on perceived functional ability and self-efficacy of elder females with arthritis.* Dissertation. University of Kansas, Lawrence, KS.

Ferrari, M. (2001, November/December). Music notes (Training tips). *American Fitness, 19,* 48-50.

Fibromyalgia definitions, facts and statistics. (2002). (Online), November 11, 2002 from Colorado Healthsite at http://www.coloradohealthsite.org/fibro/fibro_stats.html

Fibromyalgia: What's in a name? (1990, September). *Harvard Medical School Health Letter, 15,* 4-6.

Flavonoids, the next new thing. (2000, February). *Harvard Health Letter, 26,* ITEM00349004.

Gaby, A. (2001). Intravenous nutrients relieve the symptoms of fibromyalgia. *Townsend Letter for Doctors and Patients,* 14.

Gardiner, R. & Howe, C. (1998, July). Fibromyalgia and exercise. *The Backletter, 13,* 76.

Gordon, N. (1993). *Arthritis: Your complete exercise guide.* Champaign, IL: Human Kinetics Publishers.

Gorman, C & Park, A. (2002, December 9). The age of arthritis. *Time, 162,* 71-79.

Green, V. (2001). The new food pyramid. (Online), June 5, 2002 from The Tufts Daily at http://www.tuftsdaily.com/archives/Fall2001/F1003c.html

Gutfeld, G. & Sangiorgio, M. (1993, June). Bulk up the joint: Can strength training ease effects of rheumatoid arthritis? *Prevention, 45,* 16-17.

Harvard School of Public Health. (2004). Food pyramids. (Online), November 15, 2004 from http://www.hsph.harvard.edu/nutritionsource/pyramids.html

Hecht, A. (1993). Hocus-pocus as applied to arthritis: *FDA Consumer Magazine,* 1080.

Hills, M. & Horwood, J. (1994). *Exercise and arthritis: A guide to pain-free movement.* Allentown, PA: People's Medical Society.

Hoeppner, L. (1992). *The effects of water exercise versus open swim on the mood states, pain, and flexibility of older adults with osteoarthritis.* Dissertation. University of Utah, Salt Lake City, Utah.

Holman, A. & Myers, R. (2005, August). A randomized, double-blind, placebo-controlled trial of pramipexole, a dopamine agonist, in patients with fibromyalgia receiving concomitant medications. *Arthritis and Rheumatism, 52,* 2495-2505.

Horstman, J. (1999). *The Arthritis Foundation's guide to alternative therapies.* Atlanta: Arthritis Foundation.

Horstman, J. (2001, February). More than medicine. *Arthritis Today, 15,* 63-68.

Hunder, G. (1999). *Mayo Clinic on arthritis.* Rochester: Mayo Clinic.

Huskisson, E. & Donnelly, S., (1999, July). Hyaluronic acid in the treatment of osteoarthritis of the knee. *Rheumatology, 38,* 602-607.

Intensive exercise for RA. (1996, January). *The Back Letter, 11,* 2.

Jensen, S., Cram, H., & Van Duser, B. (2000, January). Effect of music tempo on heart rate and perceived exertion during rest, exercise and recovery. *Research Quarterly for Exercise and Sport, 71,* A-29.

Jetter, J. & Kadlec, N. (1985). *Arthritis book of water exercise.* New York: Holt, Rinhart and Winston.

Johnston, K. (1992). *The effects of exercise on standing balance, pain, and coping resources maintenance: A comparison of land and water exercise for arthritis patients.* Dissertation. Georgia State University, Atlanta, GA.

Katz, D. (2002). *The way to eat.* Naperville: Sourcebooks Inc.

Kelly, D. (1993). *Aquaerobics, sr.: Easy pool exercises for seniors.* Key Largo: Top of the Mountain Publishing.

Kjeldse-Kragh, J., Haugen, M., Borchgrevink, C., Laerum, E., Eek, M., Mowinkel, P., Hovi ,K., & Forre O. (1991, July 13). Controlled trial of fasting and one-year vegetarian diet in rheumatoid arthritis. *Lancet, 338,* 85-93.

Kremer, J., Michalek, A., & Lininger, L. (1985, June 29). Effects of manipulation of dietary fatty acids on clinical manifestations of rheumatoid arthritis. *Lancet, 1,* 1471-1475.

Kubetin, S. (2002, August). Water-based exercise benefits elderly women. *Family Practice News, 32,* 10.

Langer, S. (1998, March). Arthritis: A new understanding emerges. *Better Nutrition, 60,* 32-38.

La Vecchia, C., Decarli, A., & Pagano, R. (1998, March). Vegetable consumption and risk of chronic disease. *Epidemiology 9,* 208-210.

Lewis, R. (1991, July/August). Arthritis: Modern treatment for that old pain in the joints. *FDA Consumer Magazine,* 1-7.

Linos, A., Kaklamani, V., Kaklamani, E., Kouomantaki, Y., Giziaki, E., Papazoglou, S., & Mantzoros, C. (1999, December). Dietary factors in relation to rheumatoid arthritis: A role for olive oil and cooked vegetables? *American Journal of Clinical Nutrition, 70,* 1077-1082.

Mannerkorpi, K., Nyberg, B., Ahlimen, M., & Ekdahl, C. (2002, October). Six and 24 month follow-up of pool exercise therapy and education for patients with fibromyalgia. *The Journal of Rheumatology, 31,* 306-310.

Mattey, D., Hutchinson, D., Dawes, P., Nixon, N., Clarke, S., Fisher, J., Brownfield, A., Allersea, F., Fryer, A., & Stranger, R. (2002, March). Smoking and disease severity in rheumatoid arthritis association with polymorphine at the glutathione S-Trasferase M1 Locus. *Arthritis & Rheumatism, 46,* 640-646.

McAlindon, T., Felson, D., Zhang,Y., Hannan, M., Aliabadi, P., Wissman, B., Rush, D., Wilson, P., & Jacques, P. (1996, September). Relation of dietary intake and serum levels of vitamin D to progression of osteoarthritis of the knee among participants in the Framingham Study. *Annals of Internal Medicine, 125,* 353-360.

McCook, A. (2002, September). Arthritis more common in smokers, divorced. *Journal of Rheumatology, 29,* 1981-1989.

Melton-Rogers, S., Hunter, G., Walter, J., & Harrison, P. (1996, October).

Cardiorespiratory responses of patients with rheumatoid arthritis during bicycle riding and running in water. *Physical Therapy, 76,* 1058-1065.

Meyer, B. & Lemley, K. (2000, October). Utilizing exercise to affect the symptomatology of fibromyalgia: A pilot study. *Official Journal of the American College of Sports Medicine, 32,* 1691-1697.

Meyer, C. (1991). *Community arthritis water exercise programs: A controlled study.* Dissertation. Wichita State University, Wichita, KS.

Munson, M. (1996, November). Tank heaven: Water exercise may unplug pain. (Hydrotherapy for arthritis). *Prevention, 48,* 40-41.

Nichols, D. & Glenn, T. (1994, April). Effects of aerobic exercise on pain, perception, affect and level of disability in individuals with fibromyalgia. *Physical Therapy, 74,* 327-332.

O'Brien, D. (2002, July 27). Aquatics offers freedom. (Online), September 3, 2002 from MARRTC at http://www.muhealth.org/~arthritis/articles/jul02/aquatic.html

Olofsson, P., Holmber, J., Turdsson, J., Lu, S., Akerstrom, B., & Homdahl, R. (2003, January). Positional identification of NCF1 as a gene that regulates arthritis severity in rats. *National Genetics, 33,* 25-32.

Ostapowicz, G., Fortana, R., Schiodt, F., Larson, A., Davern, T., Han, S., McCashland, T., Shakil, A., Han, J., Hynan, L., Crippin, J., Blei, A., Samuel, G., Reisch, J., & Lee, W. (2002, December). Results of a prospective study of acute liver failure at 17 tertiary care centers in the United States. *Annals of Internal Medicine, 137,* 947-954.

Panush, R., Wasner, C., Young, J., & Bilbrey, D. (1987). *Arthritis unproven remedies.* Atlanta: Arthritis Foundation.

Penninx, B., Messier, S., Rejeski, W., Williamson, J., DiBari, M., Cavazzini, C., Applegate, W., & Pahor, M. (2001, October). Physical exercise and the prevention of disability on activities of daily living in older persons with osteoarthritis. *Archives of Internal Medicine, 161,* 2309-2316.

Perlmutter, C. (1997, April). The truth about fibromyalgia. *Prevention, 49,* 86-93.

Phase II data presented on rheumatoid arthritis vaccine. (1999, November 29). *Immunotherapy Weekly,* NA.

Public health and aging projected prevalence of self-reported arthritis or chronic joint symptoms among person >65 years — United States 2005-2030. (2003, May 30). *Morbidity and Mortality Weekly Report, 52,* 489-491.

Published research studies confirm glucosamine/chondroitin benefits. (2001,

October 4). (Online), November 19, 2002 from ImmuneSupport.com Treatment & Research Information at http://www.immunesupport.com/library/prpint.cfm?ID=3125.

Rosenstein, A. (2002). *Water exercises for Parkinson's: Maintaining endurance, strength, flexibility, and balance.* Ravensdale, WA: Idyll Arbor, Inc.

Russell, I., Gilbert, A., Morgan, W., & Bowden, C. (1986, March). Is there a metabolic basis for the fibrosistis syndrome? *The American Journal of Medicine, 1986,* 50-54.

Rx for arthritis sufferers: Exercise. (1996 July). *Tufts University Diet & Nutrition Letter, 14,* 1.

Sadovsky, R. (2002, November). Hyaluronic acid cuts pain, improves knee osteoarthritis. *American Family Physician, 65,* 2354.

Santen, M. & Yeager, S. (2002, March). Arthritis relief: Add water: Aquatic exercise may make moving easier. *Prevention, 54,* 68.

Sayce, V. & Fraser, I. (1989). *Exercise can beat your arthritis.* Garden City Park: Avery Publishing Group Inc.

Schieszer, J. (2003, February). Hold the water. *Better Homes and Gardens, 81,* 239.

Science backs cod liver oil as cure for arthritis. (2002). (Online), August 12, 2003 from http://www.eurekalert.org/pub_releases/2002-02/cu-sbc022002.php

Shawe, D., Hesp, R., Gumpel, J., Smbrook, P.& Reeve, J. (1993, March 23). Physical activity as a determinant of bone conservation in the radial diaphsis in rheumatoid arthritis. *Annals of the Rheumatic Diseases, 52,* 579-581.

Sherman, C. (1992, October). Managing fibromyalgia with exercise. *The Physician and Sportsmedicine, 20,* 166-172.

Simeon, M. & Flynn, J. (1999). *The John Hopkins white papers, arthritis.* New York: Medletter Associates, Inc.

Simon, H. (Ed.). (2002, May). Aspirin and its rivals. *Harvard Men's Health Watch, 7,* 1-5.

Sobel, D. & Klein, A. (1993). *Arthritis: What exercises work.* New York: St. Martin's Press.

Stein, C. (2000). *Arthritis medicines A-Z.* New York: Random House Inc.

Stewart, M., Malkovska, V., Krishnan, J., Lesin, L., & Barth, W. (2001, September). Lymphoma in a patient with rheumatoid arthritis receiving

Methotrexate treatment: Successful treatment with Rituximab. *Annals of the Rheumatic Diseases, 60,* 892.

Strosberg, J. (1993, February). Reflections of unproven arthritis remedies. *New York Journal of Medicine, 93,* 118-119.

Study finds increased risk of heart disease in RA patients. (2001, July 1). *Biotech Week,* 5.

Summary health statistics for US adults: National health interview survey 1997. (2002, October). *Vital Health Statistics, 10,* 23.

Sverdrup, B., Kallberg, H., Bengtsson, C., Lundberg, I., Padyokov, L., Alfredsson, L., & Klareskog, L. (2005, September). Association between occupational exposure to mineral oil and rheumatoid arthritis: Results from the Swedish EIRA case-control study. *Arthritis Research & Therapy Journal, 7,* R1296-R1303.

Takeshima, N., Rogers, M., Watanabe, E., Brechue, W., Okada, A., Yamada, T., Islam, M., & Huyano, J. (2002, March). Water-based exercise improves the health-related aspects of fitness in older women. *Medicine and Science in Sports and Exercise, 33,* 544-551.

Teixeira, S. (2002, May). Bioflavonoids: Proanthocyanidins and quercetin and their potential roles in treating musculoskeletal conditions. *Journal of Orthopedic Sports Physical Therapy, 2002,* 357-363.

Van Den Ende, C. (2000, October 4). Effect of intensive exercise on patient with active rheumatoid arthritis: A randomized clinical trial. *JAMA, The Journal of American Medical Association, 284,* 1631.

Van Den Ende, C., Hazes, J., Cessie, S., Mulder, W., Belfor, D., Breedveld, F., & Dijkmans, B. (1996, November). Comparison of high and low intensity training in well controlled rheumatoid arthritis. *Annals of the Rheumatic Diseases, 55,* 798-805.

Van Tilburg, A. (1999). *The importance of verbal and nonverbal communication in teaching water aerobics.* Dissertation. The University of Toledo, Toledo, Ohio.

Vitamin A toxicity: Not as rare as you think. (1995, July). *Environmental Nutrition, 18,* 8.

Voorhees, D. (1993). *The book of totally useless information.* New York: MJF Books.

Wallace, D. (2002). *All about fibromyalgia.* Los Angeles: Oxford University Press.

Ward, A. (1999). *Aquatic therapy usage among physical therapists and athletic trainers.* Graduate Thesis. Georgia Southern University, Statesboro, GA.

Watkins, R. (1988). *The water workout recovery program.* Chicago: Contemporary Books Inc.

Welch, G. (1998, May/June). Fibromyalgia: What is it? How do we deal with it? *American Fitness, 16,* 18-22.

Westfall, J. (1999). *The effects of a water exercise program on the manifestations of fibromyalgia.* Thesis. Slippery Rock University, Slippery Rock, PA.

Whitney, L., Deel, D., Marple, J., Metzger, S., Wilder, M., & Harrison, A. (2000, May). Balance, fear of falling, and quality of life in arthritic elders participating in an aquatic exercise program. *Physical Therapy, 80,* S36.

Williamson, D. (1998, November 9). Study reveals possible link between osteoarthritis and diet. (Online), Retrieved October 26, 2003 from http://www.eurekalert.org/pub_releases/1998-11/UoNC-SRPL-091198.php

YMCA of America. (1987). *Aquatics for special populations.* Champaign, IL: Human Kinetics Publishers.

YMCA of the USA & Arthritis Foundation. (1996). *Arthritis Foundation YMCA Aquatic Program (AFYAP).* Atlanta: The Arthritis Foundation.

Index

About the Author

Ann Rosenstein has been a water and land fitness instructor since 1989. She is certified through the Aquatic Exercise Association (AEA), the Aerobics and Fitness Association (AFAA), LIFT, Schwinn Cycling, and the Physicalmind Institute. Ms. Rosenstein instructs classes in water aerobics, indoor cycling, indoor rowing, weight lifting, and Pilates for the Northwest Athletic Clubs (a division of Wellbridge Corporation). Ann is also a certified physical trainer through AFAA. She has been named instructor of the year for the Northwest Athletic Clubs three times and received their Star Excellence award for superior customer service and satisfaction.

Besides authoring *Water Exercises for Rheumatoid Arthritis*, Ann has written *Water Exercises for Parkinson's, Water Exercises for Fibromyalgia, and Water Exercises for Osteoarthritis*.

Ms. Rosenstein has a B.A. and an M.A. degree from the University of Minnesota. When not teaching fitness, she is also employed as a reference librarian. Her hobbies are music, fitness, writing, and spending time with her family.

Ann resides in Burnsville, MN with her husband Leo and their children Sarah and Ben.